Oral Pathology in the Pediatric Patient

Elizabeth Philipone · Angela J. Yoon
Ioannis G. Koutlas

Oral Pathology in the Pediatric Patient

A Clinical Guide to the Diagnosis and Treatment of Mucosal and Submucosal Lesions

Second Edition

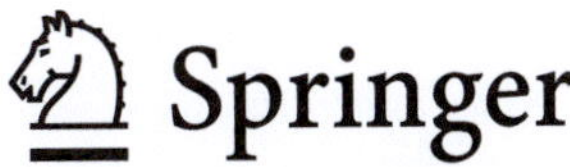

Elizabeth Philipone
College of Dental Medicine
Columbia University Irving Medical Center
New York, NY, USA

Angela J. Yoon
Oral and Maxillofacial Pathology
Medical University of South Carolina
Charleston, SC, USA

Ioannis G. Koutlas
School of Dentistry
University of Minnesota
Minneapolis, MN, USA

ISBN 978-3-031-30902-1   ISBN 978-3-031-30900-7   (eBook)
https://doi.org/10.1007/978-3-031-30900-7

This Springer imprint is published by the registered company Springer Nature Switzerland AG
The registered company address is: Gewerbestrasse 11, 6330 Cham, Switzerland

Preface

All three authors of *Oral Pathology in the Pediatric Patient: A Clinical Guide to the Diagnosis and Treatment of Mucosal and Submucosal Lesions* practice clinical oral pathology and are certified by the American Board of Oral and Maxillofacial Pathology. Based on their experiences seeing patients and supervising active biopsy services, they have compiled a sampling of the oral mucosal lesions most likely to be encountered in everyday practice. The authors' goal was to create an easy-to-use reference guide for clinicians to turn to for guidance in identifying and managing the more frequent oral mucosal lesions presenting in pediatric patients.

Oral mucosal lesions are not uncommon in the pediatric population. Fortunately, the vast majority of mucosal lesions are benign, and many are transient—being of either a traumatic or infectious etiology. Often a diagnosis can be rendered by coupling a careful clinical history with the clinical presentation.

For each entity covered in this manual, characteristic clinical photographs are provided, the clinical appearance is concisely described, and guidance is offered on formulating a differential diagnosis and selecting appropriate treatment.

Oral mucosal indications of systemic diseases, clinical indicators of drug use, sexual abuse, and eating disorders are addressed in Chap. 2.

For those lesions in which the clinical diagnosis and subsequent patient management is unclear, it is best to seek a second opinion from a specialist. In addition, it is also often prudent to communicate your findings to the child's pediatrician. Having a complete and accurate medical history is crucial for proper patient management.

New York, NY, USA   Elizabeth Philipone
Charleston, SC, USA   Angela J. Angela
Minneapolis, MN, USA   Ioannis G. Koutlas

Acknowledgments

We would like to express our sincere thanks to Drs. David Zegarelli, Michael Z. Marder, Robert J. Gorlin, Carl Witkop, Heddie O. Sedano, and Robert A. Vickers, for providing clinical photographs and for sharing their vast clinical experience and knowledge with us.

We would like to extend a special thank you to Dr. Andrea Mann, pediatric dentist, Basking Ridge, NJ, for sharing her wealth of experience and expertise in caring for pediatric patients.

Contents

Part I   Mucosal and Submucosal Lesions

1   Mucosal and Submucosal Lesions   3
  1.1   Papillary Lesions   28
  1.2   Oral Ulcers   35
  1.3   Perioral Lesions   60
  1.4   White and Red Macules and Patches   66
  1.5   Gingival Lesions   80
  1.6   Pigmented Lesions   105

**Part II   Mucosal Manifestations of Systemic Disease,
               Habits and Abuses**

2   Mucosal Manifestations of Systemic Disease, Habits and Abuses . . .   119
  2.1   Mucosal Manifestations of Gastrointestinal Disease   119
  2.2   Mucosal Manifestations of Nutritional Deficiencies   123
  2.3   Mucosal Manifestations of Immunosuppression   126
  2.4   Oral Manifestations of Habits and Abuse   130
  2.5   Oral Soft Tissue Manifestations of Hematologic Disorders   136
       2.5.1   White Blood Cell Disorders   136
       2.5.2   Red Blood Cell Disorders   141
       2.5.3   Platelet Disorders   141

Part III   Sample Cases

3   Diagnoses and Management   145

References   155

Index   157

Part I

Mucosal and Submucosal Lesions

Mucosal and Submucosal Lesions

Mucosal and submucosal lumps and bumps are more accurately referred to as nodules. In general, mucosal and submucosal nodules do not spontaneously resolve and often require surgical excision for precise diagnosis and treatment. A retrospective analysis of 3,129 oral pathology biopsy specimens from pediatric patients (0–18 years of age) submitted for diagnosis to Columbia University Medical Center, Department of Oral and Maxillofacial Pathology found mucocele and fibroma to comprise the two most frequently diagnosed soft tissue lesions. In this chapter, we review the clinical appearance, etiology, differential diagnosis, and recommended treatment for some of the more commonly encountered submucosal nodules encountered in the pediatric population.

Gingival nodules are covered in Sect. 1.4.

Mucosal nodules
Mucocele
Fibroma
Pyogenic granuloma
Hemangioma
Lymphangioma
Peripheral nerve sheath lesions (e.g., Neurofibroma and mucosal neuroma)[a]

[a]Not common, but presents in children and can be the initial presentation of Neurofibromatosis, Multiple endocrine neoplasia syndrome, type IIB, and as manifestations of *PIK3CA* Related Overgrowth Spectrum

Mucocele

Clinical appearance: Smooth-surfaced soft tissue mass/bump that often has a slightly bluish hue. Mucoceles vary in size from a few millimeters to a few centimeters. Some patients might report that the lesion increases and decreases in size. They are often asymptomatic. The surface can appear ulcerated if the child chews or habitually bites it.

Etiology: Trauma resulting in the spillage of mucin into the connective tissues.

E. Philipone et al., *Oral Pathology in the Pediatric Patient*,
https://doi.org/10.1007/978-3-031-30900-7_1

Location: Anywhere salivary glands are located; the *lower lip* is the most common location.

Differential diagnosis: Salivary duct cyst, salivary gland tumor, fibroma, pyogenic granuloma, benign connective tissue tumor (i.e., lipoma and neuroma).

Treatment: Surgical excision of the lesion together with adjacent minor salivary gland lobules. It is important to inform the patient and parent/guardian that the lesion can recur if re-traumatized (or if the offending/damaged salivary gland is not removed). When removing a lower lip mucocele a lateral incision should be made to avoid transecting the labial artery. Excision can also be performed using a soft tissue laser. Over 20% of mucoceles of the ventral surface of the tongue recur (personal observation). This relatively higher recurrence rate is because the associated minor salivary glands (glands of Blundin-Nuhn) are embedded within skeletal muscle and their harvesting/excision can be challenging.

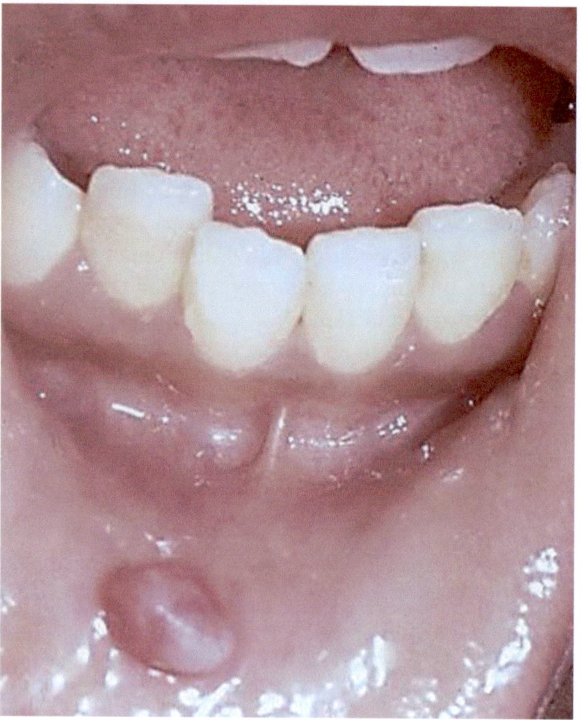

Fig. 1.1 Mucocele. Raised pink nodule of the lower lip

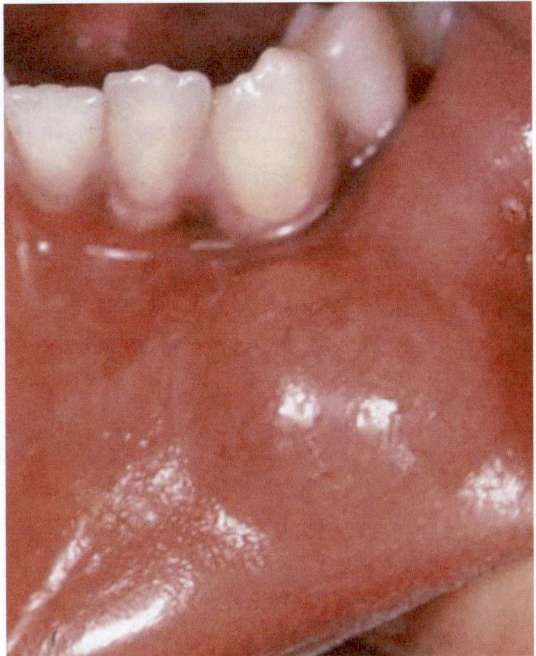

Fig. 1.2 Mucocele. Submucosal nodule of the lower lip

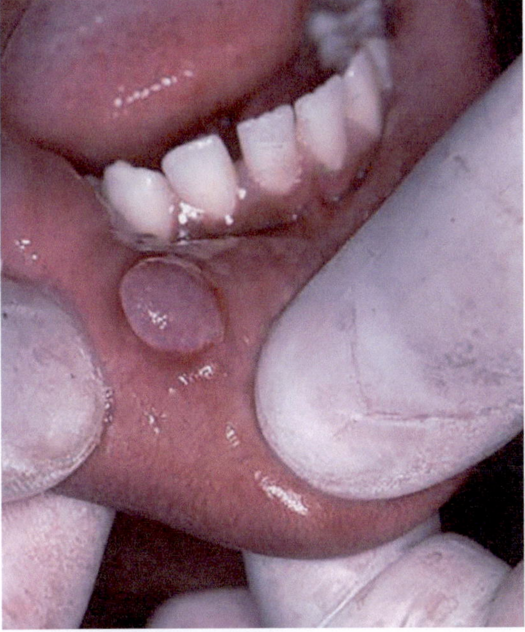

Fig. 1.3 Mucocele. Raised pink, semi-translucent nodule of the lower lip

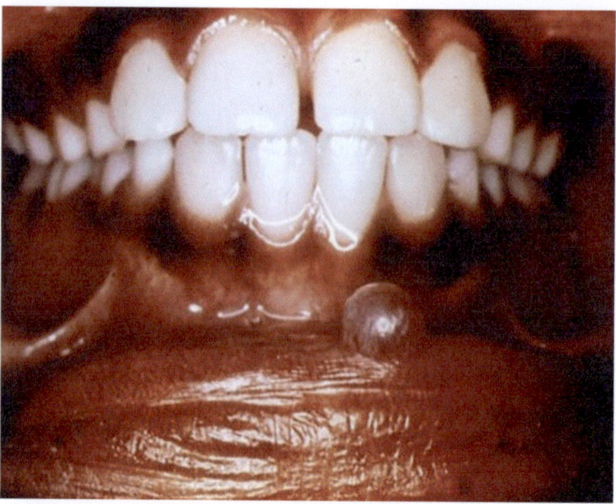

Fig. 1.4 Mucocele. Raised semi-translucent nodule of the lower lip

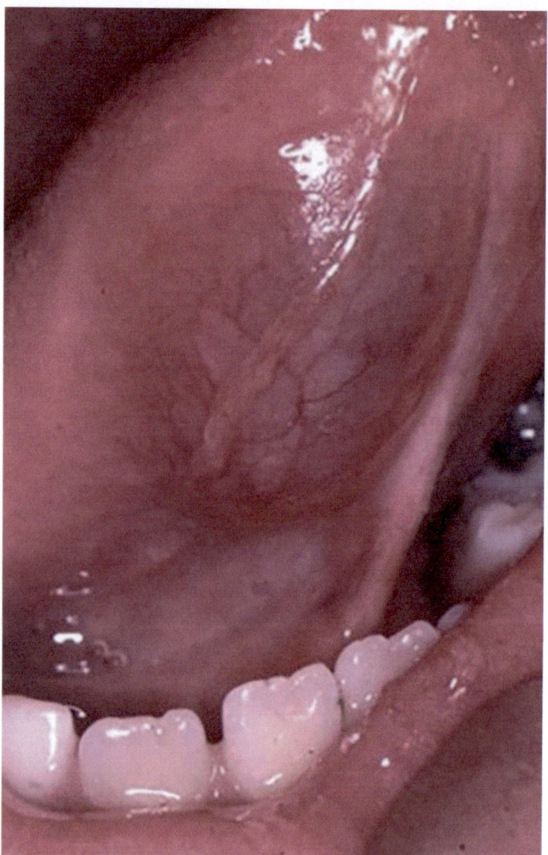

Fig. 1.5 Mucocele. Submucosal swelling of the ventral tongue

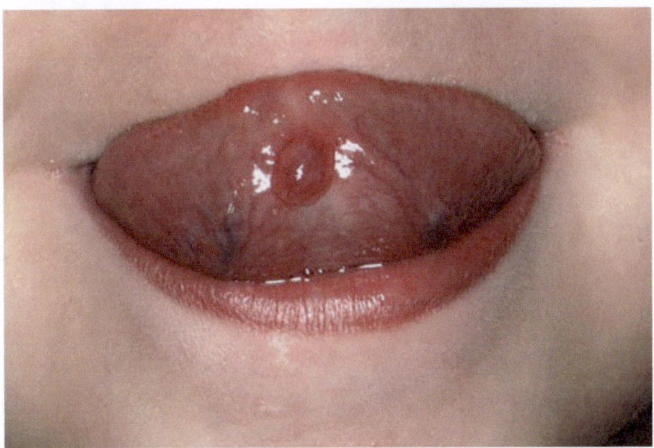

Fig. 1.6 Mucocele. Mucocele of ventral tongue

Ranula

A ranula is a mucocele of the floor of the mouth involving the sublingual gland or possibly the submandibular gland (less often). Ranulas are most common in children and young adults.

Clinical appearance: Smooth-surfaced soft tissue mass/swelling occurring on the floor of the mouth, lateral to the midline. Ranulas often have a slightly light bluish hue and can reach several centimeters. The lesion can increase and decrease in size. The child might complain of discomfort or be asymptomatic.

Etiology: Trauma or obstruction of one of the ducts of the sublingual gland or of the submandibular duct.

Location: Floor of mouth, lateral to the midline.

Differential diagnosis: Salivary gland tumor, dermoid cyst, abscess.

Treatment: If caused by obstruction from a sialolith (salivary duct stone), removal of the stone can be curative. Sialoliths, however, are more frequently encountered in adult patients. Otherwise, surgical excision of the ranula together with the feeding gland is the definitive treatment. A less invasive approach is to de-roof the ranula and allow the tissue to granulate. However, with this approach, the lesion may recur.

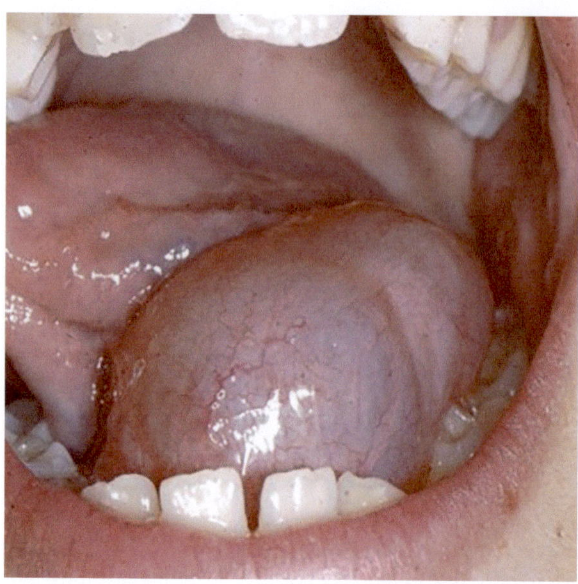

Fig. 1.7 Ranula. Fluctuant submucosal mass of the left floor of the mouth causing tongue displacement

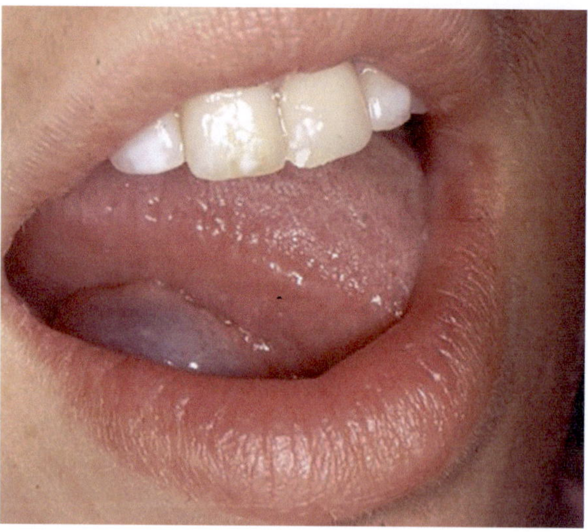

Fig. 1.8 Ranula. Submucosal mass of the left floor of mouth

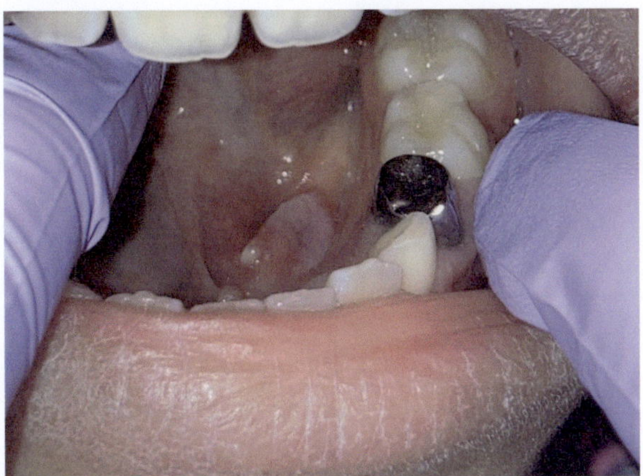

Fig. 1.9 Deflated ranula of the floor of the mouth of a 10-year-old female. History of recurrent episodes of enlargement

Clinical Clue Ranulas occur lateral to midline. A submucosal floor of mouth mass occurring at the midline and resulting in elevation of the tongue is more likely a dermoid cyst (See Fig. 1.14).

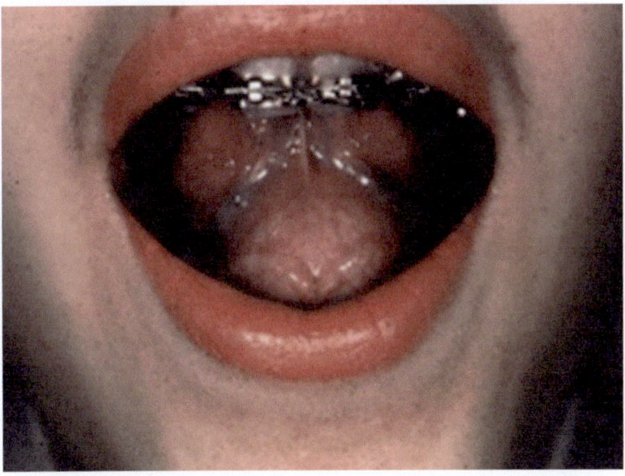

Fig. 1.10 Dermoid cyst. Note the location at the midline as opposed to the lateral presentation of the ranulas shown in Figs. 1.7, 1.8, and 1.9

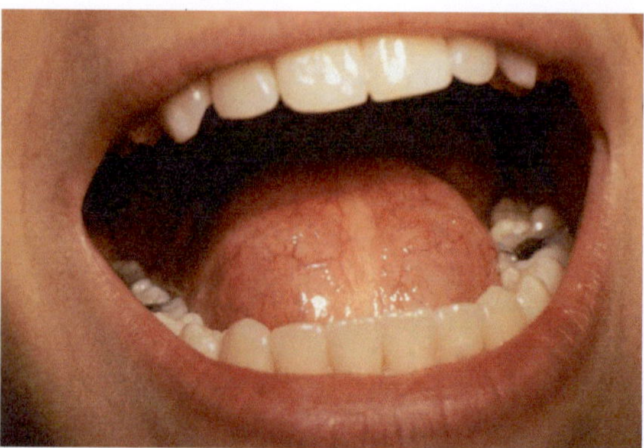

Fig. 1.11 Dermoid cyst. Large, midline, submucosal swelling of midline floor of mouth cuasing superior displacement of the tongue

Plunging Ranula

A plunging ranula is a ranula which extends below the mylohyoid muscle into the neck, presenting as a painless, recurrent, or progressive lateral neck swelling. Most also have an intraoral component.

The *differential diagnosis* for a plunging ranula includes congenital lymphatic or vascular anomalies such as cystic hygroma, cervical abscess (usually associated with a carious tooth), cystic or necrotic lymph node, thyroglossal duct cyst (usually midline), brachial cleft cyst (usually at the anterior border of sternocleidomastoid muscle). Imaging studies can be helpful in confirming a clinical diagnosis of plunging ranula and to identify the feeding gland.

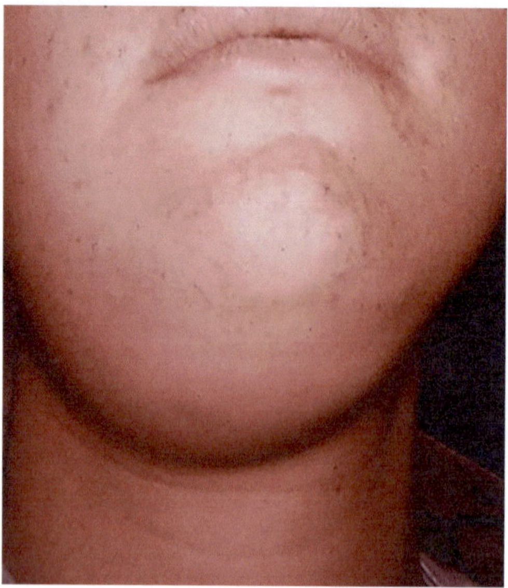

Fig. 1.12 Plunging ranula. Unilateral submandibular swelling

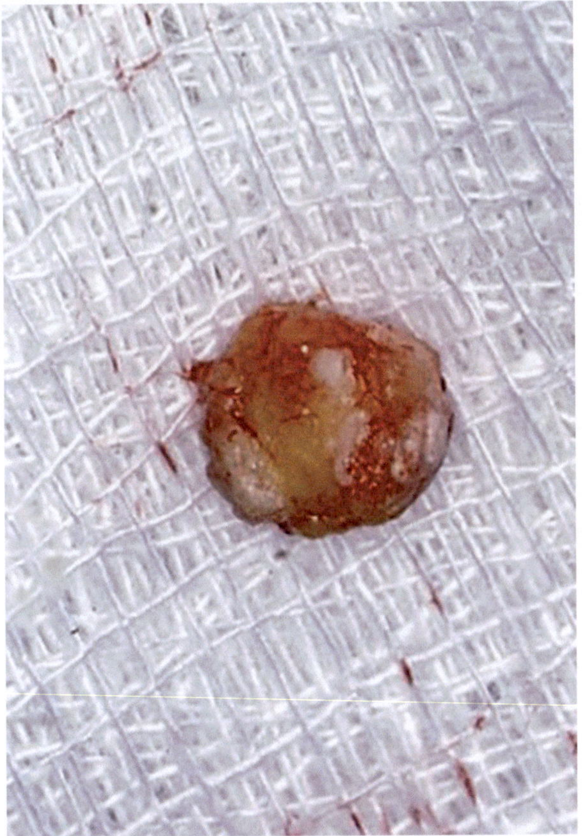

Fig. 1.13 Sialolith. *Sialoliths* appear as yellow-tan round to ovoid stones

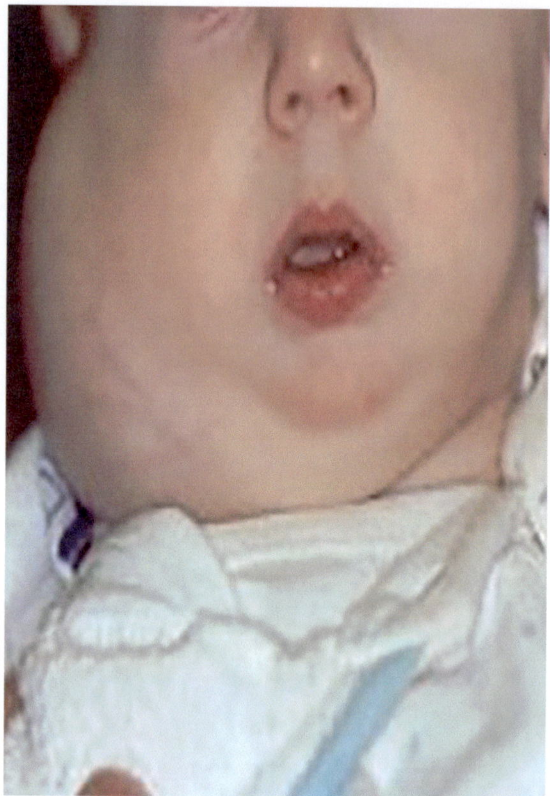

Fig. 1.14 Cystic hygroma. Large cystic swelling of the right neck in an infant

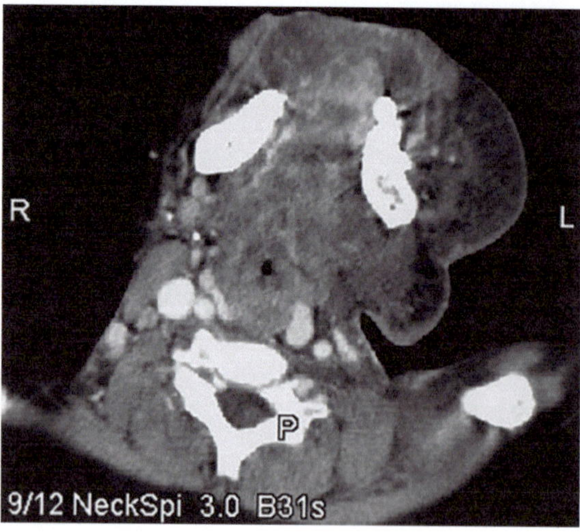

Fig. 1.15 Cystic hygroma, CT, axial image. Fluid filled cytic structiure of the left side of the neck infiltrating the laryngeal wall and causing stenosis of the larynx

Salivary Gland Tumors

Less than 5% of salivary gland tumors occur in children and adolescents. In children and adolescents, the incidence of benign versus malignant salivary gland tumors is similar. As in adults, pleomorphic adenoma is the most common benign tumor in children and mucoepidermoid carcinoma is the most common malignant. In general, the parotid gland is the most common site for salivary gland tumors, followed by the intraoral minor salivary glands. Intraoral salivary gland tumors present as a submucosal swelling or mass. In some cases, the clinical appearance can be essentially similar to a mucocele. Painless swelling is the main presentation of both benign and malignant salivary gland tumors. The presence of surface ulceration can raise the suspicion of malignancy. Benign salivary gland tumors are treated by excision which is frequently curative. Malignant salivary gland tumors are most often treated surgically. It is suggested, however, to be managed by a multidisciplinary pediatric oncology team.

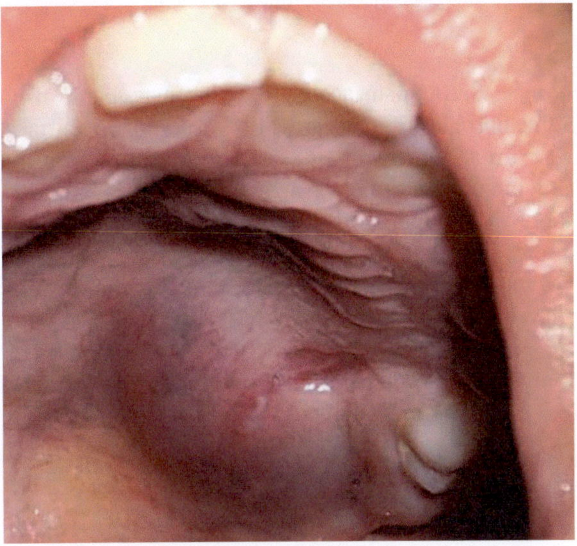

Fig. 1.16 Mucoepidermoid carcinoma. Asymptomatic palatal swelling in an 11-year-old girl. Biopsy revealed a low-grade mucoepidermoid carcinoma

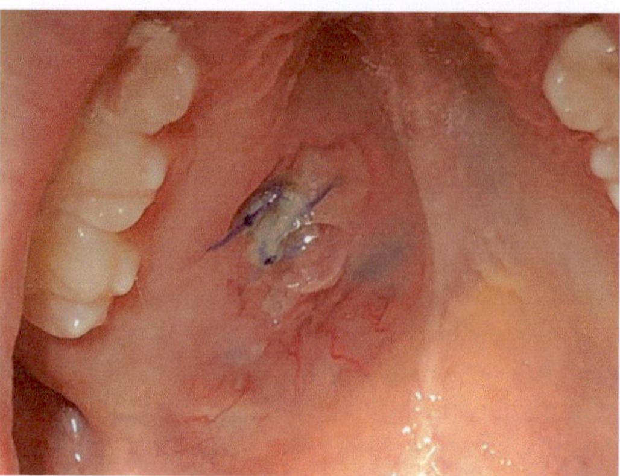

Fig. 1.17 Mucoepidermoid carcinoma. Ulcerated palatal swelling in a child. Photo taken post-biopsy. Biopsy revealed a low-grade mucoepidermoid carcinoma

Fibroma

Clinical appearance: Smooth-surfaced soft tissue mass/bump that is sessile and pink in color. Some fibromas can appear whitish as a result of surface keratinization caused by chronic irritation (i.e., biting). Sometimes the surface can be ulcerated. Fibromas are slow-growing and vary in size from a few millimeters to a few centimeters. They are often asymptomatic.

Etiology: Chronic irritation or chronic trauma, i.e., cheek biting.

Location: Anywhere, often in locations easily exposed to chronic irritation such as the buccal mucosa or lower lip.

Differential diagnosis: Mucocele, pyogenic granuloma, neuroma, lipoma, papilloma.

Treatment: Surgical excision, recurrence unlikely unless chronic irritation continues (i.e., cheek biting habit).

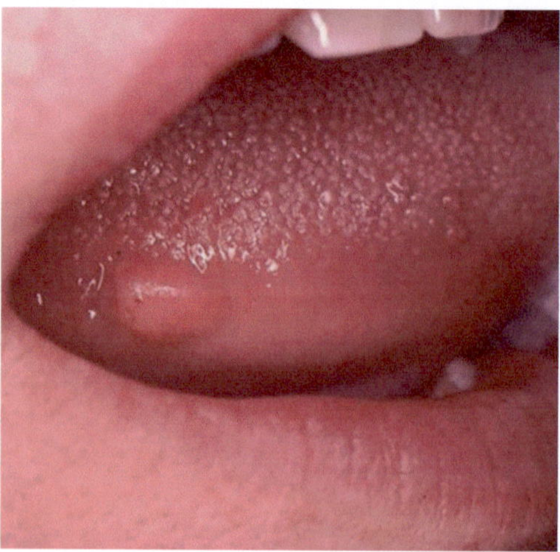

Fig. 1.18 Fibroma. Pink sessile exophytic nodule of the lateral tongue

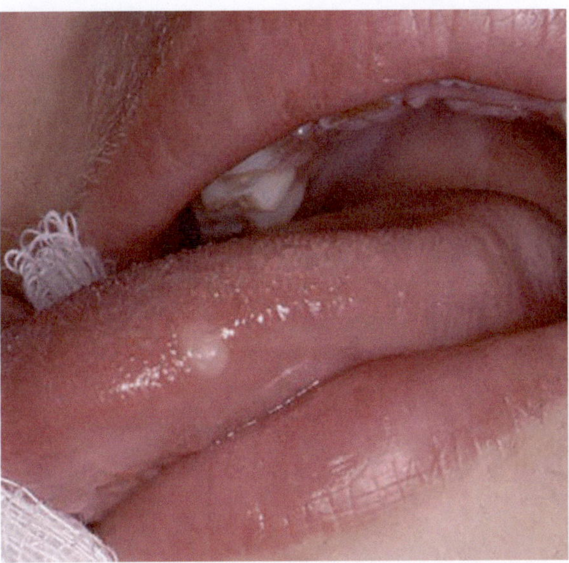

Fig. 1.19 Fibroma. Pink-white sessile exophytic nodule of the lateral tongue. Fibromas can sometimes appear slightly whitish. This is due to excess keratin production resulting from chronic irritation, i.e., biting

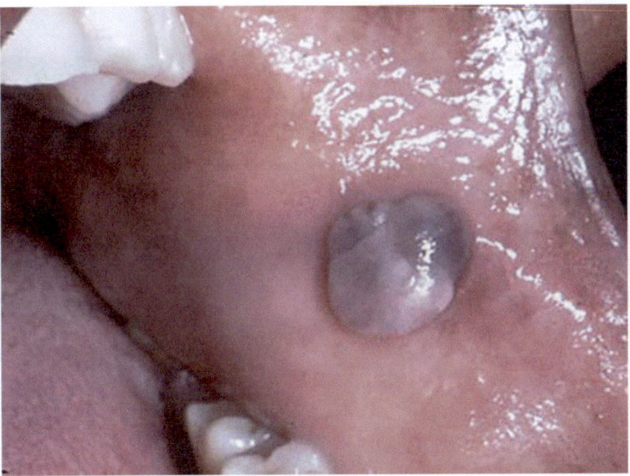

Fig. 1.20 Fibroma. Exophytic nodule of the anterior buccal mucosa with a partial purplish hue. This may have been the result of secondary hemorrhage from biting. Based on color the differential diagnosis could include a pyogenic granuloma or mucocele. Also note the faint physiologic pigmentation near the border adjacent to the lip

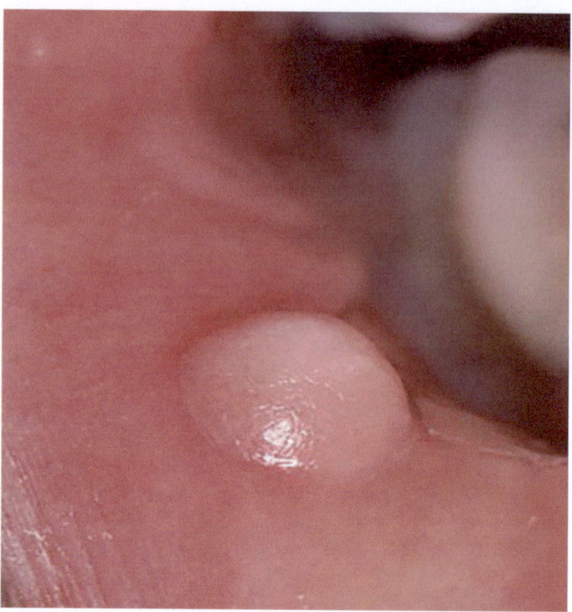

Fig. 1.21 Fibroma. Pink-white exophytic nodule of the lower labial mucosa

Pyogenic Granuloma

Sometimes histologically referred to as a *lobular capillary hemangioma*.

Clinical appearance: Smooth-surfaced soft tissue mass/bump that often has a red appearance. Often bleeds when manipulated. The surface may or may not be ulcerated. Can vary in size, most often a few to several millimeters. Often asymptomatic.

Etiology: Excess granulation tissue formation—often resulting from local irritation (i.e., plaque accumulation) or from trauma.

Location: Anywhere in the oral cavity, the gingiva is the most common site.

Differential diagnosis: Fibroma, mucocele, hemangioma, peripheral ossifying fibroma (if on gingiva), peripheral giant cell granuloma (if on gingiva).

Treatment: Surgical excision, recurrence is possible.

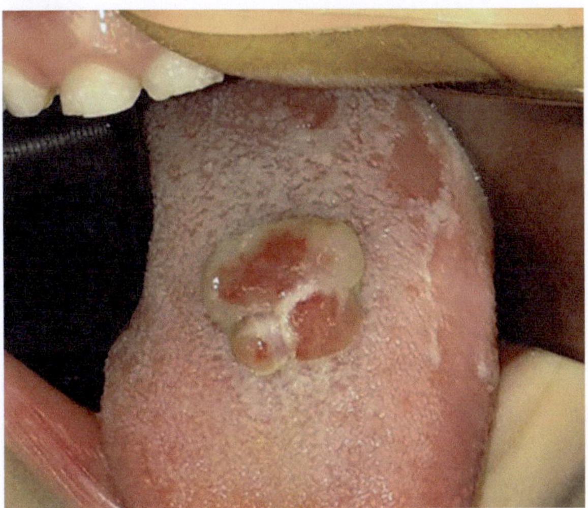

Fig. 1.22 Pyogenic granuloma. Lobular tan-red exophytic nodule of the dorsal tongue of a 6-year-old child with history of injuring her tongue with a Popsicle stick. Note the child also has benign migratory glossitis (geographic tongue). Photo courtesy of Dr. David Koslovsky, New York, NY

Hemangioma

Clinical appearance: Smooth-surfaced soft tissue mass or swelling with a red or purplish-blue hue.

Etiology: Benign tumor of endothelial cells which typically appears in the first weeks of life, grows rapidly over the first 6 months, stabilizes, and gradually involutes. Involution can take several years.

Location: Anywhere, the tongue is a common location.

Differential diagnosis: Vascular malformation, hematoma, pyogenic granuloma, mucocele.

Treatment: Most hemangiomas disappear without treatment. If the hemangioma interferes with eating, speaking, or breathing, or it is of significant cosmetic concern, treatment can be rendered. Treatment options include sclerotherapy—the injection of a sclerosing agent such as propranolol, intralesional corticosteroid, and IV vincristine, the latter for large and life-threatening lesions. Surgical removal is a less commonly used option.

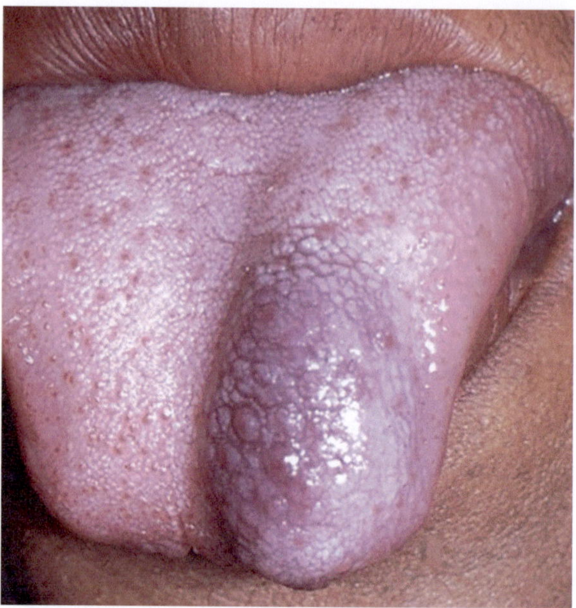

Fig. 1.23 Hemagioma. Purplish submucosal mass of the left anterior tongue present since infancy. Growth of the lesion was commensurate with growth of patient. The lesion was non-pulsatile and demonstrated blanching

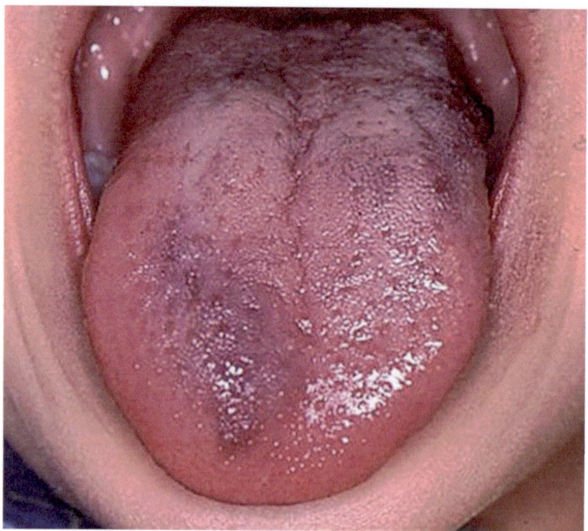

Fig. 1.24 Hemagioma. Non-pulsatile purplish submucosal mass of the tongue present since infancy. The lesion blanched when pressure was applied

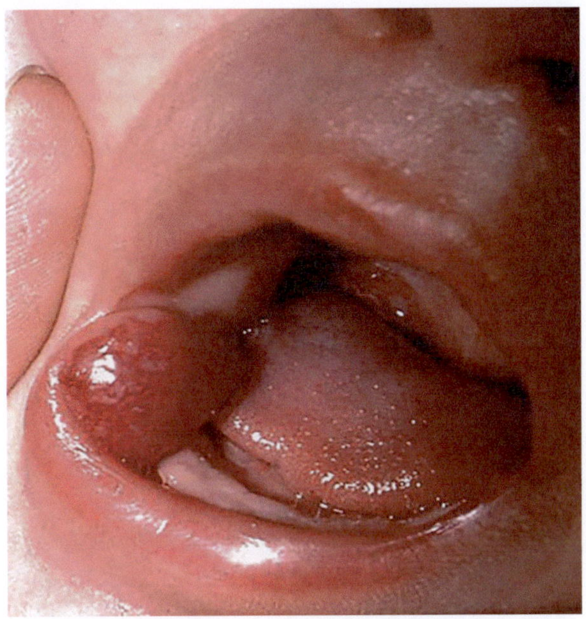

Fig. 1.25 Hemangioma. Red, non-pulsatile exophytic mass of the lower labial and anterior buccal mucosa in an infant. Blanching was noted

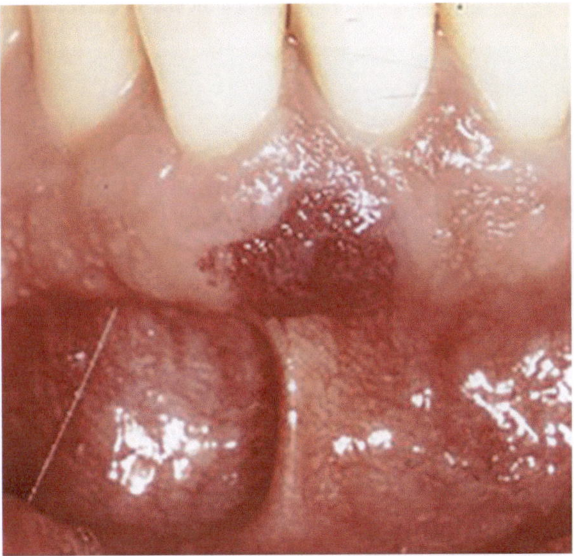

Fig. 1.26 Hemangioma. Flat, red, non-pulsatile patch of the lower facial attached gingiva in an adolescent. Blanching was noted

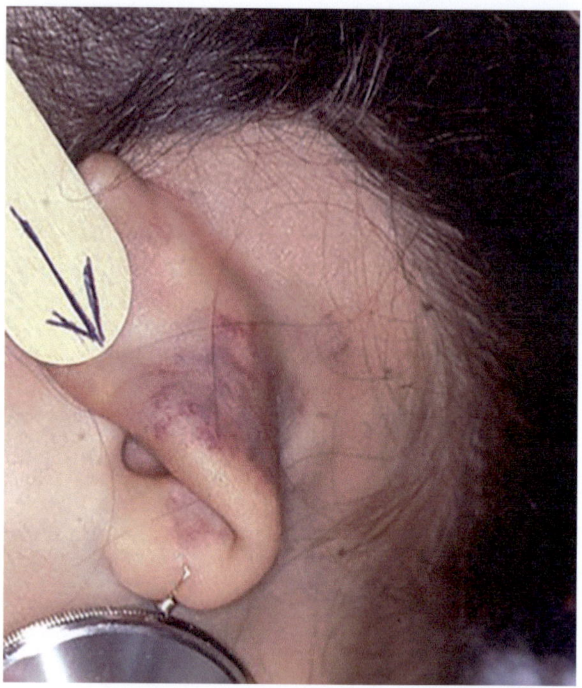

Fig. 1.27   Hemangioma of the auricular and posterior auricular skin in a child

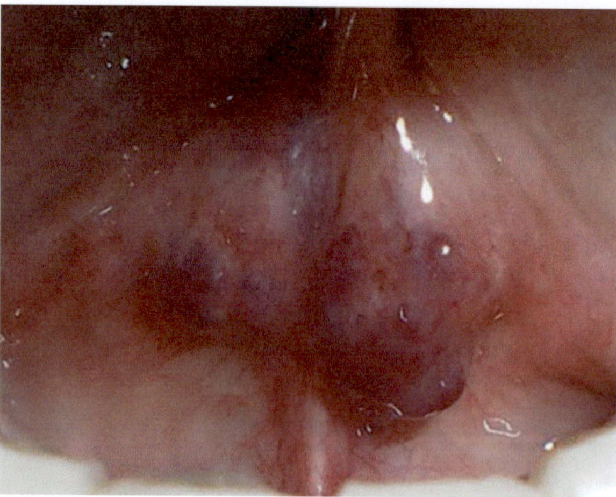

Fig. 1.28   Hemangioma. Purple lobular appearing submucosal mass of the ventral tongue in the location of the lingual frenum

Lymphangioma

Lymphangiomas are lymphatic malformations with a predilection for the head and neck. About half of all cases are congenital. Most of the remaining half manifest before age two.

Clinical appearance: The most frequent oral location is the tongue which can result in macroglossia. Superficial lesions result in the appearance of tiny blebs—so-called *frog spawn* or *caviar tongue*. Occasionally, the vascular abnormality is a combination of hemangioma and lymphangioma. Lesions in the neck are referred to as cystic hygromas and present as fluctuant masses that can become rather large.

Etiology: Benign tumor-like proliferation of lymphatic vessels.

Location: Anywhere, especially common in the head and neck, the tongue is the most common oral site.

Differential diagnosis: Hemangioma, vascular malformation, mucosal neuromas.

Treatment: Dependent on size and location. Treatment ranges from observation to surgical excision to sclerotherapy.

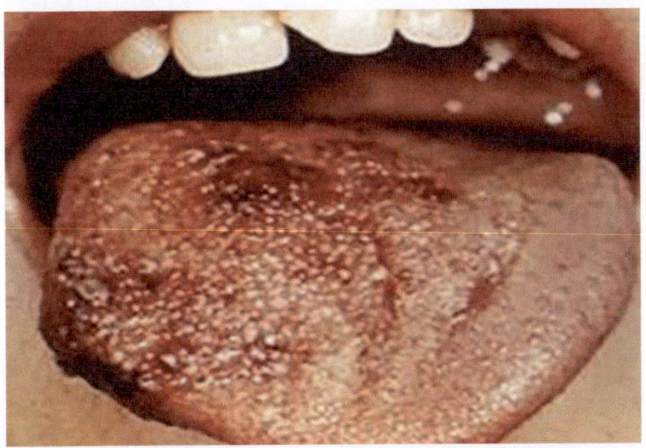

Fig. 1.29 Lymphangioma. Macroglossia with a pebbled and focally purple surface to the dorsal tongue. The purple color might be the result of secondary hemorrhage

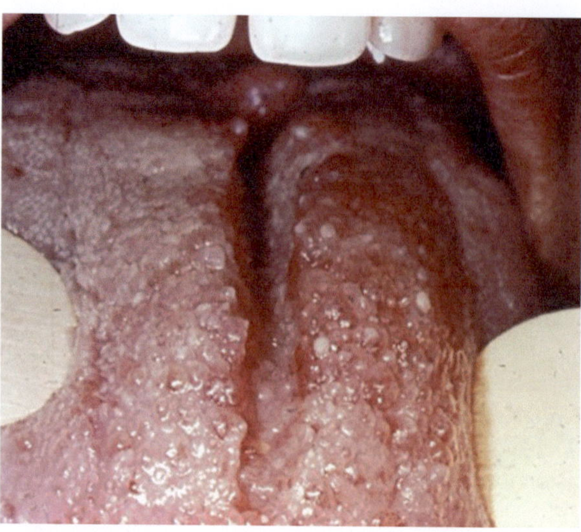

Fig. 1.30 Lymphangioma. Raised pebbly appearance of the dorsal tongue composed of small vesicles which are said to resemble caviar or fish eggs

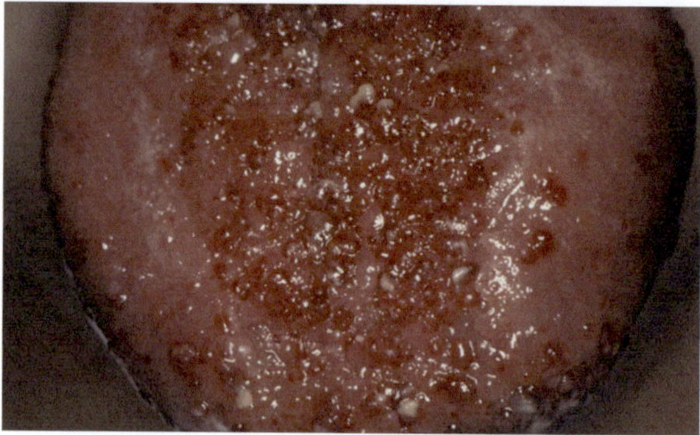

Fig. 1.31 Lymphangioma. Numerous red/pink and focal white small papules of the dorsal tongue resulting in a pebbled appearance

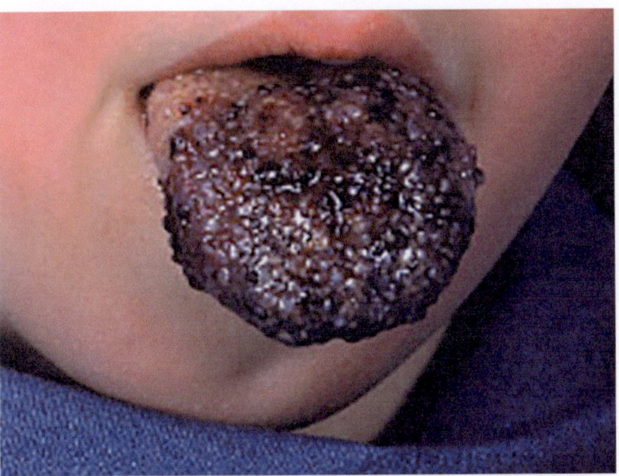

Fig. 1.32 Hemangiolymphangioma. Raised pebbly appearance of the dorsal tongue composed of small, dark vesicles. *Hemangiolymphangioma* is a rare, mixed malformation containing both vascular and lymphatic elements

Vascular Malformation

Unlike hemangiomas—which often regress with time, vascular malformations are *persistent*. This developmental condition is present at birth and represents structural anomalies of blood vessels. Vascular malformations can be either high flow (arteriovenous malformation) or low flow (capillary or venous malformations). A classic example of low-flow capillary malformation is a facial port-wine stain which may or may not be associated with Sturge-Weber Syndrome.

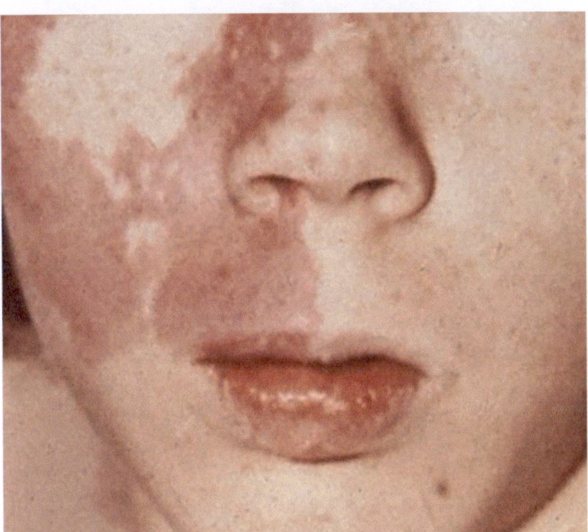

Fig. 1.33 Facial port-wine stain. Red patch of the facial skin in a child. The lesion was present since birth

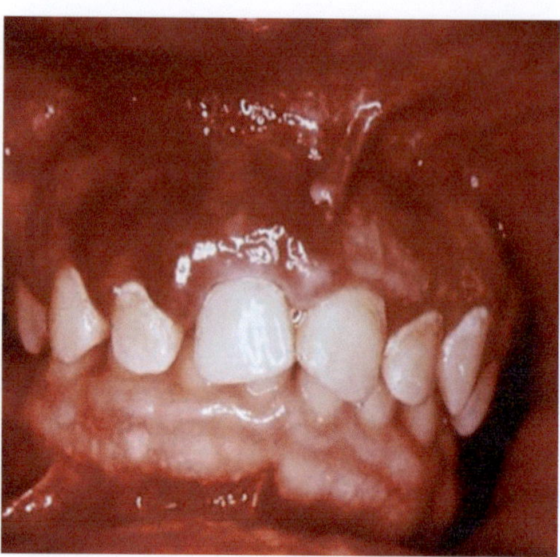

Fig. 1.34 Vascular malformation. Intraoral photo of child in Fig. 1.33. The vascular malformation involved the underlying the gingiva and labial mucosa. The tissue appeared erythematous and bulbous. Blanching was noted

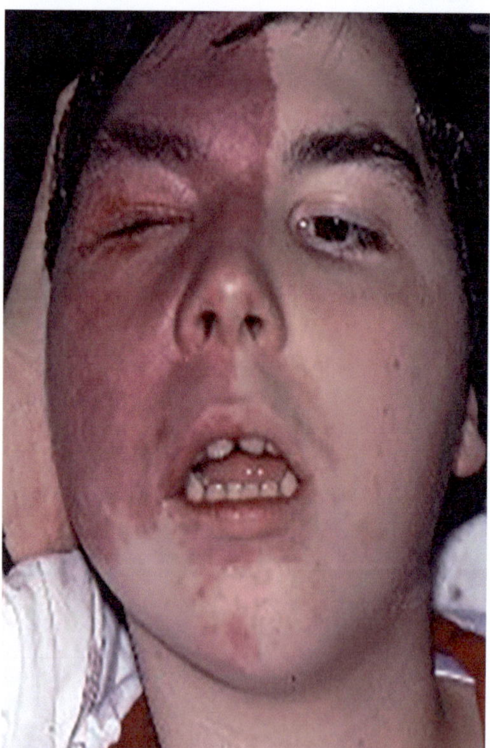

Fig. 1.35 Vascular malformation. Photograph of an adolescent with Sturge-Weber syndrome with facial port-wine stain

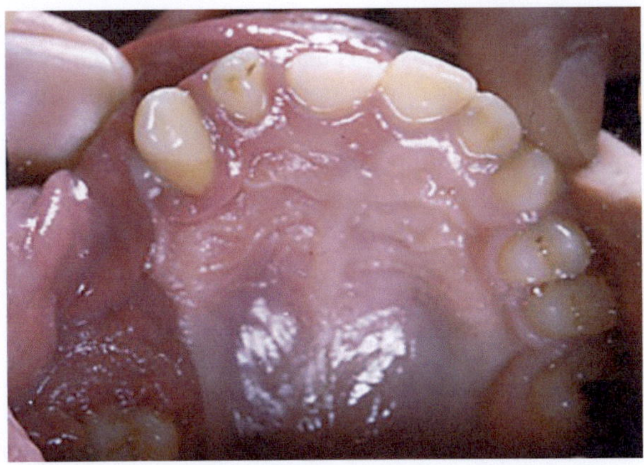

Fig. 1.36 Vascular malformation involving maxillary gingiva adjacent to facial port-wine stain

Clinical Clue To confirm the vascular nature of the lesion you can apply gentle pressure to test for *blanching*. A pulse can be detected in high-flow vessels. Also, remember hemangiomas and AV-malformations appear in infancy, thus, history of onset of the lesion is helpful.

Note Performing surgery on a lesion supplied by a high-flow vascular malformation can be dangerous, possibly even fatal, unless proper precautions are taken such as pre-operative embolization after vascular imaging.

Neural Lesions

Neural lesions of the oral cavity include neurofibroma, traumatic neuroma, solitary circumscribed neuroma, schwannoma, and mucosal neuroma. The specific type of neural tumor is significant since some are characteristic of particular genetic syndromes. Etiology is dependent on the particular type of lesion. The etiology of a traumatic neuroma is not surprisingly, trauma. The other neural lesions are considered benign tumors or hyperplasias. With the exception of mucosal neuroma, neural lesions are more commonly encountered in adults. Therefore, the below information will be restricted to *mucosal neuromas*.

Mucosal Neuromas

Clinical appearance: Smooth-surfaced soft tissue nodule or submucosal mass, typically multiple. The tongue, lips, and buccal mucosa, particularly the commissure areas are common locations. Mucosal neuromas are a distinctive feature of multiple endocrine neoplasia type 2B (aka MEN3). Other manifestations of MEN2B include skeletal anomalies, i.e., marfanoid habitus, high-arched palate, broad foreheads, and hypertelorism. Multiple submucosal neuromas of the conjunctiva and eyelids are also frequent and pathognomonic of MEN2B.

Etiology: Mucosal neuromas are benign nerve tumors of multiple endocrine neoplasia type 2B (aka MEN3). MEN2B is an autosomal dominant genetic syndrome also characterized by the frequent occurrence of medullary thyroid cancer (MTC) and pheochromocytoma.

Location: Anywhere, tongue, lips, and buccal mucosa, particularly the commissure bilaterally, are common locations.

Differential diagnosis: Traumatic fibroma(s), neurofibroma(s), Heck's disease.

Treatment: Biopsy to establish the diagnosis. Surgical excision is indicated only for lesions that are bothersome.

Besides MEN2B, patients with segmental orofacial overgrowth as part of the *PIK3CA*-related overgrowth spectrum (PROS) can present with neuromatous lesions usually affecting the perineurial envelope or just enlarged peripheral nerves that, microscopically, are indistinguishable from MEN2B. Clinicopathologic correlation and genetic testing can differentiate the two entities. Of interest is that some of these patients present with enamel hypoplasia or congenitally missing teeth/arrested development of teeth.

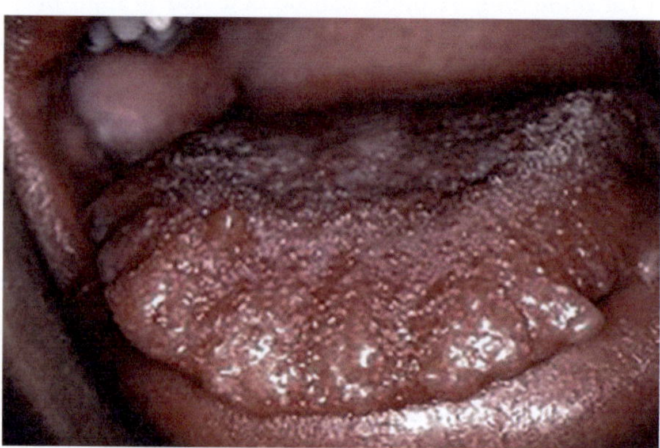

Fig. 1.37 Mucosal Neuromas. Multiple exophytic and submucosal nodules presenting in a patient with MEN2B

Mucosal neuromas can be the earliest notable manifestation of MEN2B and thus the dentist can play a pivotal role in diagnosing the syndrome. Early diagnosis of MEN2B is critical, due to the high incidence of medullary thyroid carcinoma which typically develops early in life.

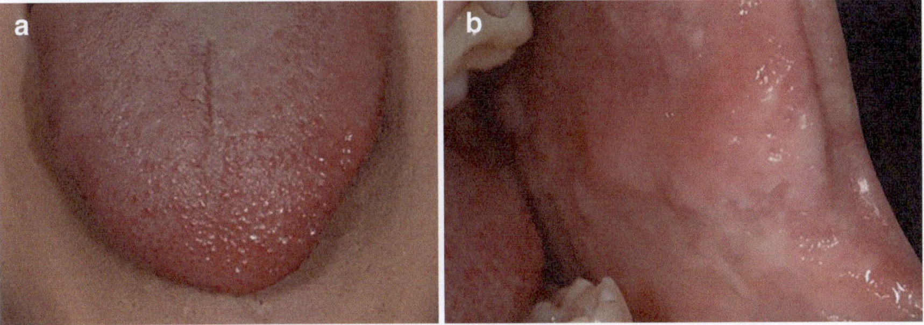

Fig. 1.38 (**a, b**) Mucosal Neuromas. Multiple, subtle, submucosal nodules presenting in a patient with MEN2B

A Note on Soft Tissue Sarcomas

Soft tissue sarcomas are rare malignant soft tissue tumors that can initially present as a painless mucosal nodule or swelling. However, as opposed to benign soft tissue tumors—sarcomas behave aggressively, typically demonstrating rapid growth. Soft tissue sarcomas comprise approximately 3% of all childhood tumors. *Rhabdomyosarcoma* is the most common soft tissue sarcoma of childhood and most often involves the head and neck region. Approximately 10% of cases are seen in oral cavity. The most common oral site is the tongue, followed by the palate and buccal mucosa. Biopsy is required to differentiate rhabdomyosarcoma from other aggressive childhood diseases such as synovial sarcoma, lymphoma, and alveolar soft part sarcoma.

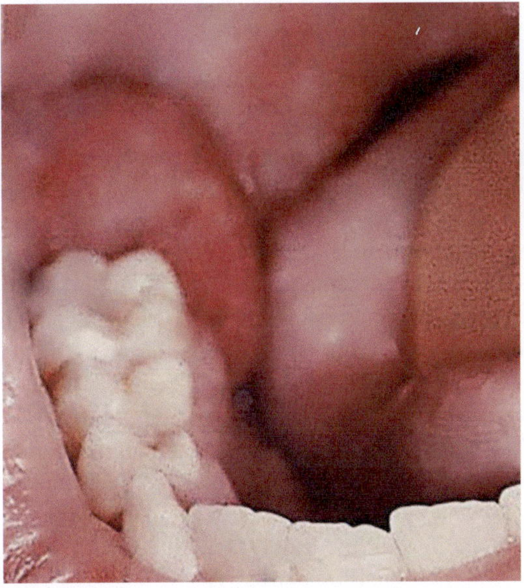

Fig. 1.39 Rhabdomyosarcoma. Painless soft tissue mass of retromolar pad

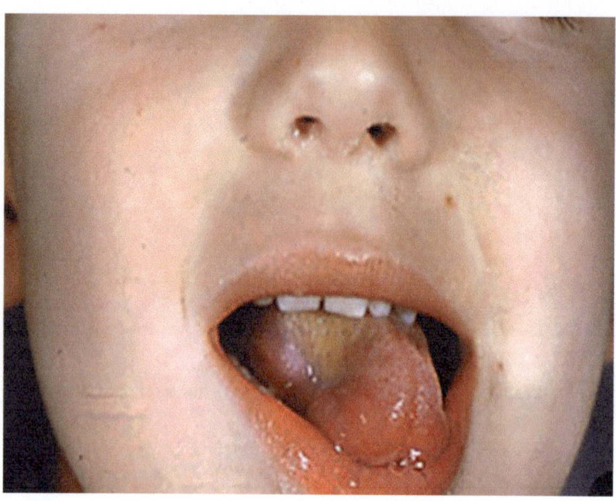

Fig. 1.40 Rhabdomyosarcoma. Firm submucosal mass of the right tongue

Clinical Note Any lesion demonstrating aggressive clinical behavior—such as rapid growth should be viewed as suspicious and further evaluation is mandated.

1.1 Papillary Lesions

Papillary Lesions
Verruca vulgaris
Squamous papilloma
Condyloma
Multifocal Viral Epithelial Hyperplasia (Heck's Disease)

A variety of papillary lesions affect the oral mucosa. In this section, we will be focusing on papillary lesions caused by various subtypes of the human papillomavirus (HPV). HPV is a DNA virus that infects epithelial cells of the skin and mucosa resulting in solitary or multifocal epithelial lesions. Differentiating these lesions can be clinically difficult, in the following pages we present subtle clinical clues that can help. In some cases, histologic examination and HPV subtyping are needed to differentiate the lesions.

Verruca Vulgaris

Also known as the common skin wart. It is uncommon in mouth, but verruca vulgaris is very common on the skin, often occurring on the hands of children.

Clinical appearance: Papillary, exophytic, white growth. Vary in size, most often a few millimeters to 1 cm. Multiple lesions are not uncommon. Asymptomatic.

Etiology: Viral—human papillomavirus (HPV). The associated HPV subtypes are that of the "low-risk" subtypes (HPV-2, HPV-4, and HPV-40).

Location: Anywhere, common in the anterior aspects of the oral cavity (i.e., anterior gingiva, lips, and anterior tongue)—often the result of autoinoculation by putting infected finger(s) in the mouth.

Differential diagnosis: Squamous papilloma, condyloma acuminatum, Heck's disease, giant cell fibroma, verruciform xanthoma.

Treatment: Conservative surgical excision with recurrence unlikely. Some lesions resolve spontaneously over time.

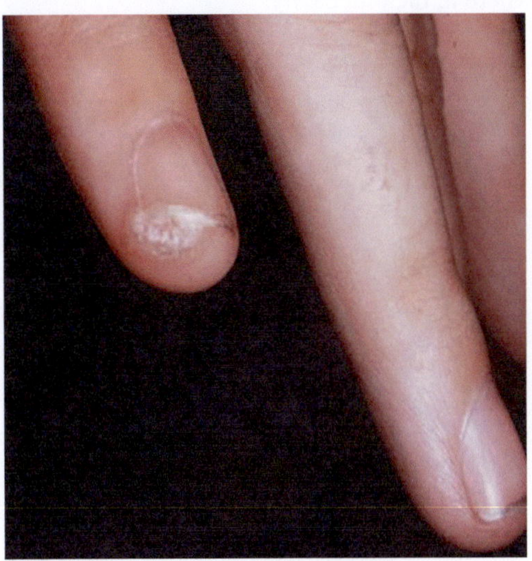

Fig. 1.41 Verruca vulgaris. White warty lesion of the fingertip and nail bed of a child

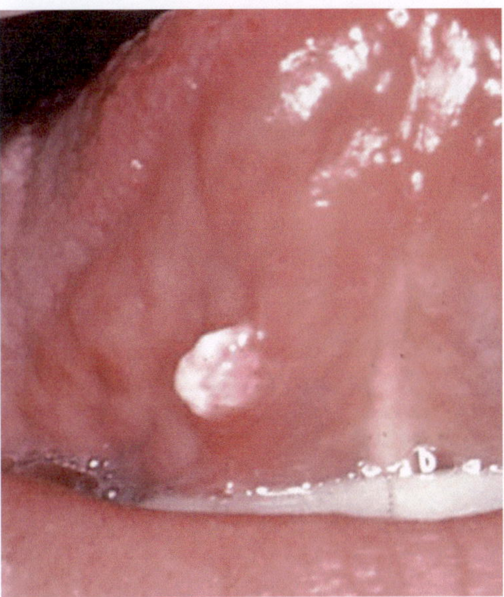

Fig. 1.42 Verruca vulgaris. White, raised, papillary growth of the ventral tongue

Clinical Clue   Examining the patient's hands for cutaneous lesions aids in diagnosis.

Squamous Papilloma

Clinical appearance: Papillary, exophytic, white growth, often on a stalk. Vary in size, most often a few millimeters to 1 cm. Most often lesions are solitary and asymptomatic.

Etiology: Viral—human papilloma virus (HPV).

Location: Anywhere in the oral cavity.

Differential diagnosis: Verruca vulgaris, condyloma acuminatum, Heck's disease, giant cell fibroma, verruciform xanthoma.

Treatment: Conservative surgical excision with recurrence unlikely.

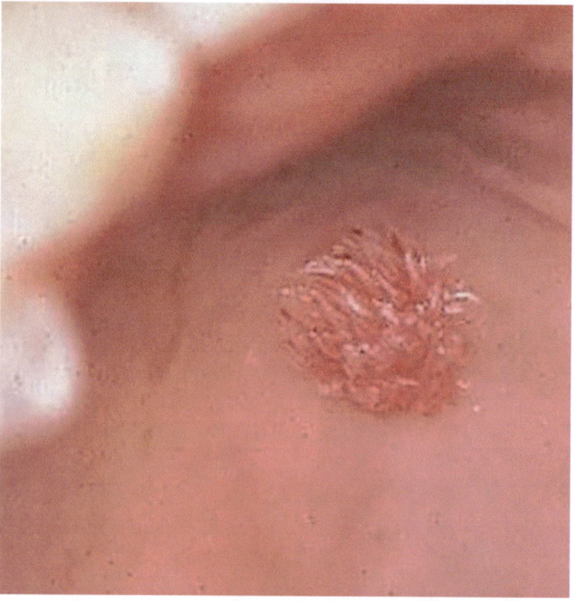

Fig. 1.43 Squamous papilloma. Exophytic growth of the anterior hard palate presenting as numerous thin pointed fronds

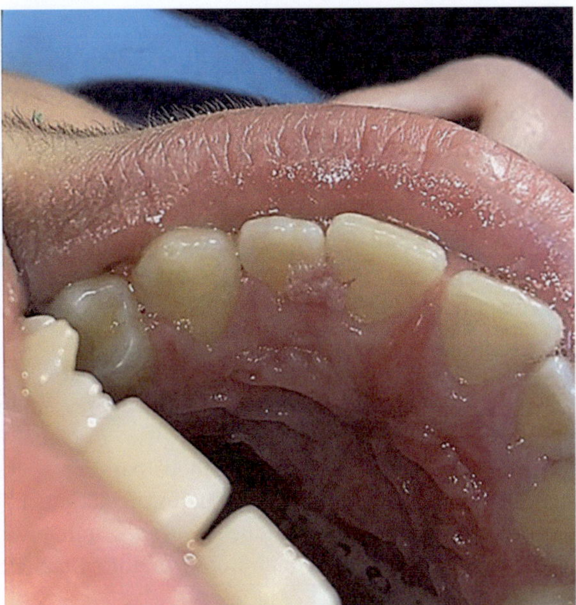

Fig. 1.44 Squamous papilloma. Pedunculated growth on lingual gingiva with a pink-white frond-like surface

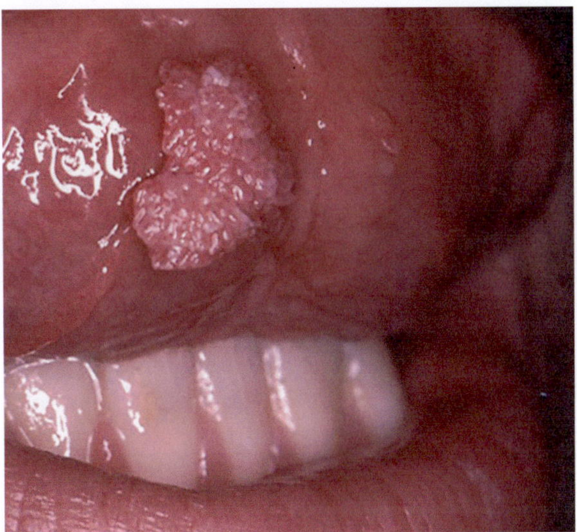

Fig. 1.45 Squamous papilloma. Exophytic growth on the lateral tongue with short white papillations. Although appearing broad, the lesion was pedunculated (stalk-like attachment)

Condyloma Acuminatum

Also known as a genital wart. It is uncommon in children. The presence of oral condylomas in children can be an indicator of *sexual abuse*.

Clinical appearance: Asymptomatic exophytic white growth with blunted papillary projections and a broad base, often described as having a cauliflower-like appearance. Condyloma vary in size but most are about 1 cm, which is larger than oral squamous papilloma and verruca vulgaris. Multiple lesions are also common.

Etiology: Viral—human papilloma virus (HPV), 90% of cases are attributed to HPV 6/11 "low-risk HPV" subtypes; however, co-infection with "high-risk" HPV subtypes 16/18 frequently occurs. Transmission can be the result of orogenital contact, prenatal infection, digital inoculation, and possibly fomite transmission. In children, sexual abuse is the most common mode of transmission.

Location: Most frequently on the soft palate, labial mucosa, and lingual frenum. The soft palate is the most common site in children.

Differential diagnosis: Verruca vulgaris, squamous papilloma, condyloma acuminatum, Heck's disease, giant cell fibroma, verruciform xanthoma.

Treatment: Conservative surgical excision, recurrence unlikely. Some lesions resolve spontaneously over time. Excisional biopsy might be required to establish the diagnosis.

> **Important Reminder**
> Suspicions of sexual abuse must be reported to the appropriate authority. The child's pediatrician should be made aware of the finding.

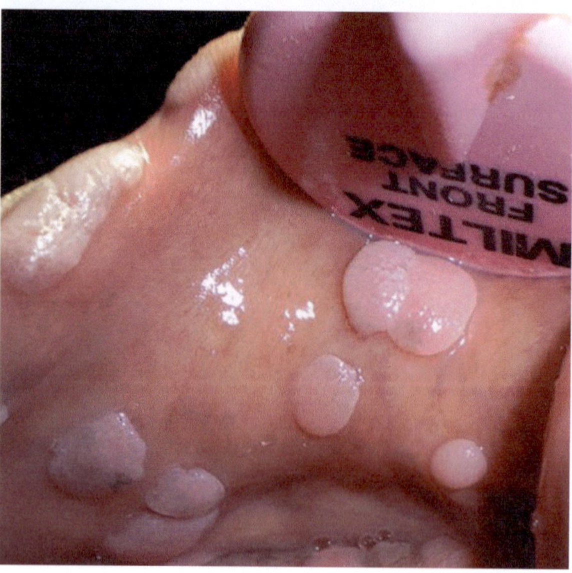

Fig. 1.46 Condyloma acuminatum. Exophytic growth of the ventrolateral tongue with short, white, blunted papillations. Patient is an adult

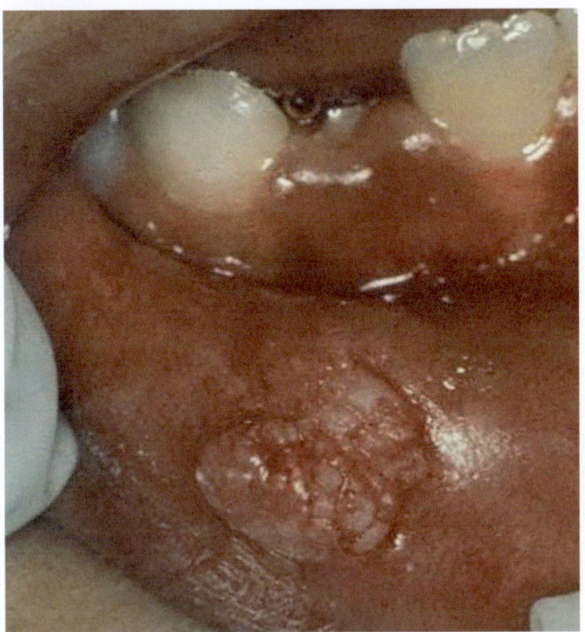

Fig. 1.47 Condyloma acuminatum. Child presenting with an exophytic growth of the lower labial mucosa. The lesion has a broad base and blunted papillations

Clinical Clue Lesions are often multiple and appear to have short blunt papillae resulting in a so-called cauliflower-like appearance. Typically, they are larger than squamous papilloma and verruca vulgaris, often occur in clusters, and have a broad base (sessile) rather than pedunculated.

Multifocal Viral Epithelial Hyperplasia (Heck's Disease)

Clinical appearance: Asymptomatic broad-based, slightly elevated, papillary or smooth-surfaced papules. The color ranges from normal mucosa to white. Individual lesions are 0.3–1.0 cm and well demarcated, but they frequently cluster together producing a cobblestone appearance. Early references report frequency among Latin American and North American Natives but it is now known that the condition can be seen in all ethnic groups. It occurs primarily in children, usually living under suboptimal hygiene and lower economic conditions. It is highly contagious.

Etiology: Viral—human papilloma virus (HPV), "low-risk" HPV subtypes 13 and 32.

Location: Anywhere in the oral cavity—sites of greatest involvement include lips, buccal mucosa and tongue.

Differential diagnosis: Verruca vulgaris, squamous papillomas, condyloma acuminatum, neurofibromas, mucosal neuromas.

Treatment: Often unnecessary. Most lesions resolve spontaneously over time (months to years). Conservative surgical excision can be performed if visible lesions are of esthetic concern. For persistent lesions, keratinolytic agents can be used with caution. Excisional biopsy might be required to establish the diagnosis.

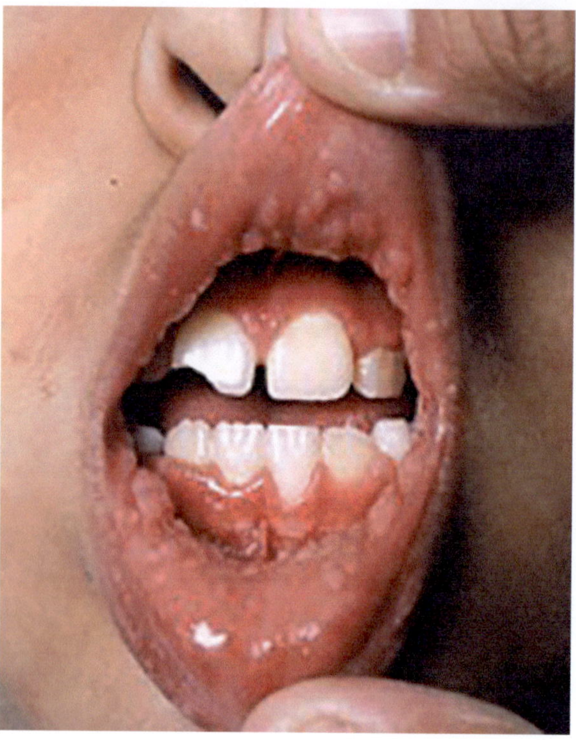

Fig. 1.48 Heck's Disease. Multiple, pink, flat to slightly papillary growths of the upper and lower lip mucosa

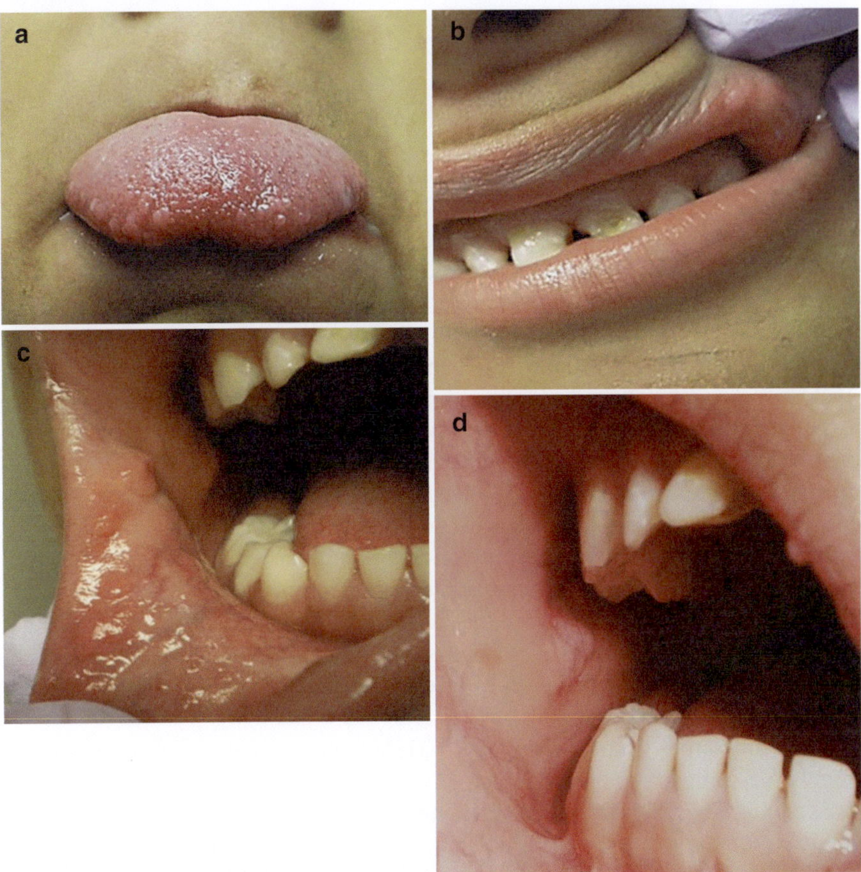

Fig. 1.49 (**a–d**) Heck's Disease. A 4-year-old South American male with multiple, pink, flat to slightly papillary growths of the anterior dorsal tongue, upper and lower lips, and buccal mucosa

1.2   Oral Ulcers

It is not uncommon to encounter ulcers in pediatric patients. Most of these ulcerations are transient and of traumatic or viral origin. Canker sores are also common in pediatric patients. The presence of persistent or continually recurring ulcers can be indications of an underlying medical condition or systemic disease (See Part II). When evaluating oral ulcerations, duration (acute vs chronic) and location (keratinized mucosa vs non-keratinized mucosa vs both) are important in determining the clinical/differential diagnosis. Chronic vesiculobullous diseases such as mucosal pemphigoid and pemphigus vulgaris are rare in children and adolescents and therefore they are not covered in this publication.

Oral Ulcerations
Viral Ulcers
   Primary Herpetic Gingivostomatitis
   Recurrent Herpetic Infection
   Herpangina
   Hand-Foot-and-Mouth disease
Non-viral ulcers
   Traumatic Ulcer
   Canker Sores
   Erythema Multiforme

Acute Herpetic Gingivostomatitis (Primary Herpes)

Acute herpetic gingivostomatitis is the symptomatic presentation of the initial exposure to the herpes simplex virus 1 (HSV-1). HSV-1 is ubiquitous and most individuals are exposed to the virus by age five. The initial infection in most patients is subclinical, however, up to 30% of children develop acute gingivostomatitis. It develops approximately one week after initial contact with an infected, often asymptomatic child or adult.

Clinical appearance: Oral lesions consist of numerous tiny vesicles, which rupture rapidly to form painful irregular ulcerations covered by yellow–gray membranes. Submandibular lymphadenitis, halitosis, and refusal to eat and/or drink are often accompanying findings. The lesions typically appear after about 3–4 days of prodromal symptoms, i.e., fever (>38 °C (100.4 °F)), anorexia, irritability, malaise, sleeplessness, and headache.

Etiology: Herpes simplex virus type 1 (HSV-1) in vast majority, rare cases result from herpes simplex virus type 2.

Location: The lesions involve both keratinized and non-keratinized mucosa. The gingiva is almost always involved—often appearing inflamed and painful.

Differential diagnosis: Erythema multiforme, recurrent aphthous stomatitis.

Treatment: Mild lesions typically heal without scarring in about a week, but healing can take up to 14–21 days in severe cases. Treatment consists of palliative care—including maintaining fluid intake and good oral hygiene. Refusal to drink can result in dehydration, which is the most frequent complication. Topical anesthetics (i.e., viscous lidocaine) and a mouth rinse containing Benadryl and Kaopectate as a rinse and spit or can be applied to the lesions using a couple of cotton swabs. OTC children's Tylenol can also be helpful. Topical anesthetics must be used with caution in children. This is due to the potential for overdose and or allergic reaction.

Medication Warning

Viscous lidocaine has a black box warning for children younger than 3 years due to reports of seizures, cardiopulmonary arrest, and death when not given per dosing and administration recommendations. Therefore, it is prudent to avoid prescribing viscous lidocaine to patients under 3 years of age.

If the child is immunocompromised or if the child is less than 6 months of age, the patient's pediatrician should be notified.

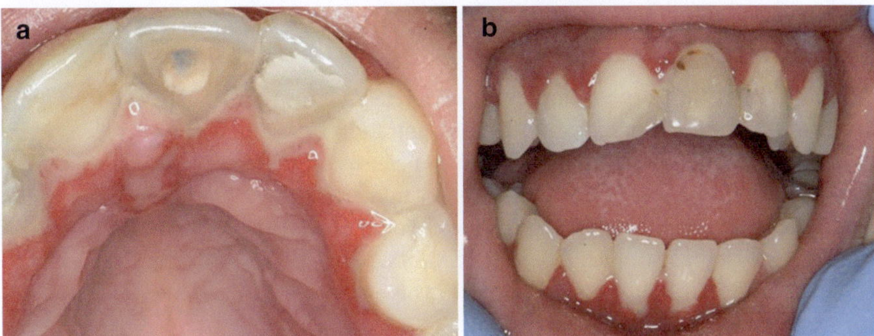

Fig. 1.50 (**a**, **b**) Primary herpetic gingivostomatitis. Fourteen-year-old presented with a 3-day duration of painfully inflamed gingiva and coalescing irregular ulcerations of the attached gingiva and anterior hard palate. Patient also had a sore throat and low-grade fever. Lesions resolved by the following week with only palliative care

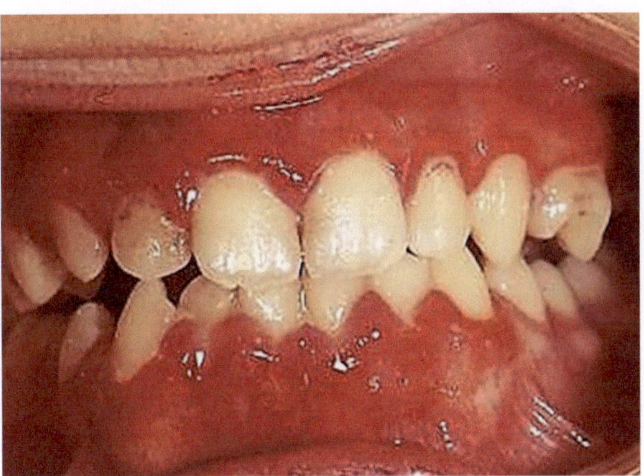

Fig. 1.51 Primary herpetic gingivostomatitis. 5-year old with painful, enlarged, and erythematous gingiva

Clinical Question: Should an antiviral medication be prescribed for a patient with primary herpetic gingivostomatitis?

Answer: Antiviral medications are most effective when taken at the onset of symptoms. Typically, when a patient with primary herpes presents to the dentist he/or she has already had the lesions for a few days. Therefore, antiviral medications are typically not prescribed. Exceptions would be if the patient is very young or immunocompromised and in those cases it is best to consult with the patient's pediatrician.

Recurrent Intraoral Herpes

Reactivation of the herpes simplex virus 1 (HSV-1) in a previously exposed child can result in intraoral or extraoral lesions. Intraoral recurrent herpes involves keratinized tissue, often the hard palate, and can cause discomfort.

Clinical appearance: Lesions consist of numerous tiny vesicles, which rupture rapidly to form small ulcers. Lesions are covered by yellow–gray membranes.

Etiology: Herpes simplex virus 1 (HSV-1).

Location: Recurrent intraoral herpes involves the keratinized mucosa only (palate, attached gingiva).

Differential diagnosis: Herpetiform aphthae, trauma, other viral ulcers.

Treatment: Lesions typically heal without scarring in about a week.

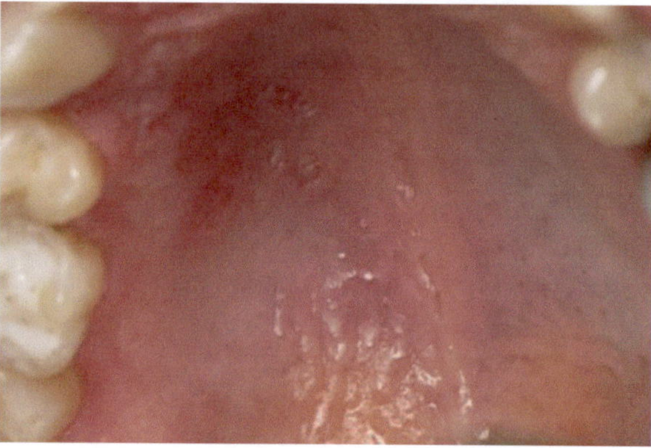

Fig. 1.52 Recurrent intraoral herpes. Multiple punctate ulcers which have begun to coalesce affecting the hard palate

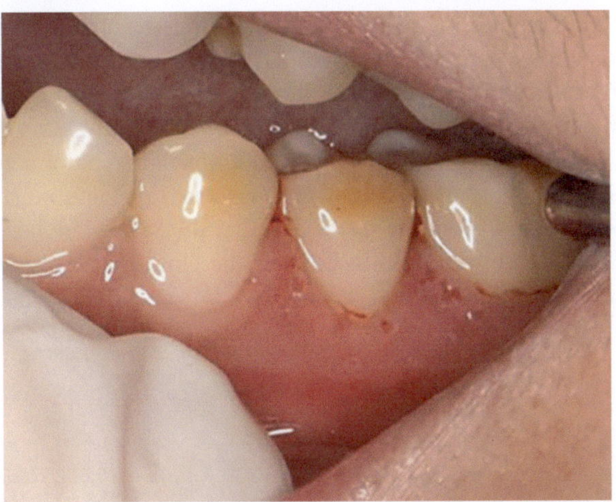

Fig. 1.53 Recurrent intraoral herpes. Multiple punctate ulcers of the attached (keratinized) gingiva

> **Reminder**
> Dental treatment can cause reactivation of the herpes virus and it is not uncommon for intraoral recurrent herpes to occur within 3 days of a dental procedure. The intraoral lesions typically occur on the palate or gingiva adjacent to the teeth which were worked on.

Herpangina

Herpangina is a highly contagious, symptomatic, self-limiting, and viral infection. Patients present with sudden high fever, sore throat, headache, neck pain, and loss of appetite. Oral lesions affecting the posterior oral cavity form within 2 days of onset of symptoms. Most cases occur in the summer and fall, affecting mostly infants and young children. It occasionally occurs in adolescents and adults. Typically spreads via the fecal-oral route or by respiratory droplets.

Clinical appearance: Few in number (often <6) 1–2 mm red macules or grayish plaques form on the soft palate and tonsillar pillars. The lesions start as vesicles that subsequently ulcerate, resulting in shallow ulcers, 2–4 mm in size with surrounding erythema, resembling oral aphthae.

Etiology: Most often Coxsackie virus A, can also be caused by Coxsackie virus B or Echoviruses.

Location: Most often soft palate and/or tonsillar pillars, can occur on the uvula, or tongue.

Differential diagnosis: Aphthous stomatitis, strep throat, other viral infections (i.e., hand foot and mouth disease, varicella-zoster, primary herpes, and mononucleosis).

Treatment: Herpangina is self-limiting and lesions resolve in less than 7 days. Antiviral medications are not effective. Treatment consists of supportive care including maintenance of fluid intake. Eating popsicles can also help soothe a sore throat. Topical anesthetics (i.e., viscous lidocaine) and/or a mouth rinse containing Benadryl and Kaopectate can be prescribed as a rinse-and-spit or can be applied to the lesions using a couple of cotton swabs. Viscous lidocaine must be used with caution (**see Medication Warning pg 36**). OTC children's Tylenol can also be helpful. If the child is immunocompromised or if the child is less than 6 months, the patient's pediatrician should be notified.

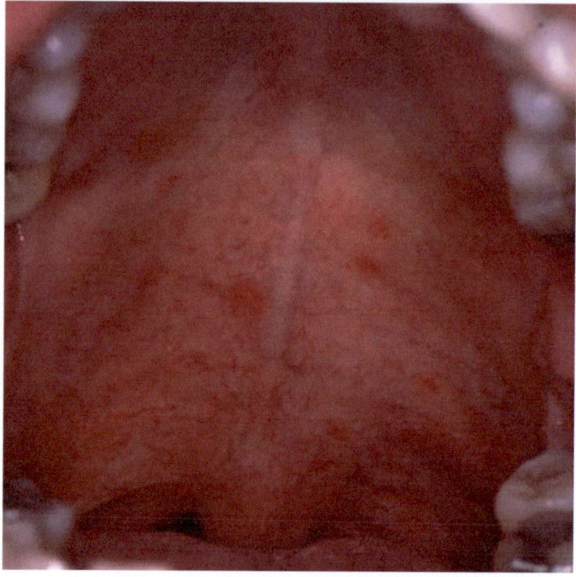

Fig. 1.54 Herpangina. Several 1–2 mm red macules of the soft palate, which will form vesicles that ulcerate

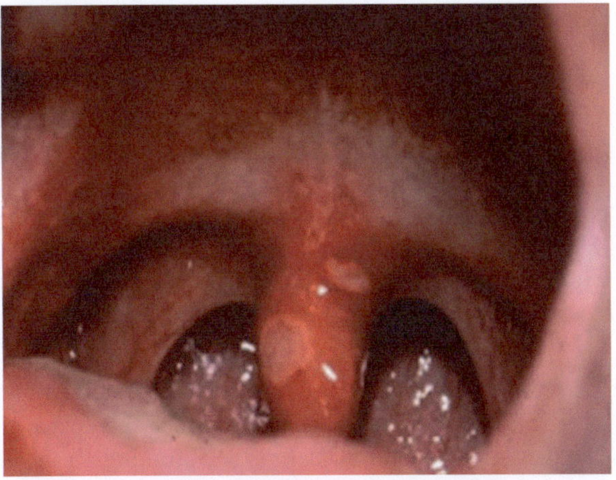

Fig. 1.55 Herpangina. Shallow, aphthous-like ulcers of the uvula and soft palate

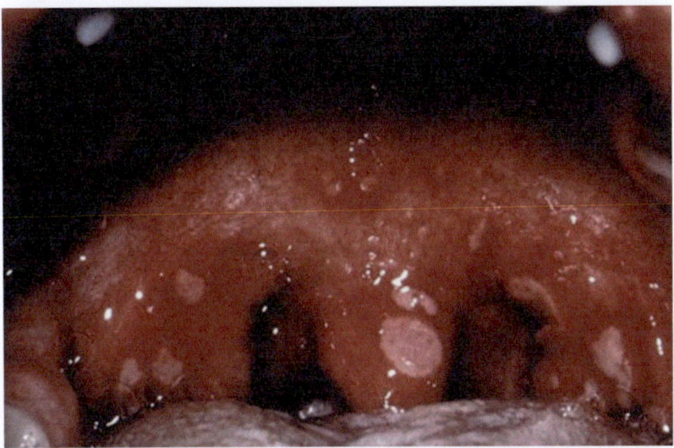

Fig. 1.56 Herpangina. Multiple shallow ulcers of the uvula, soft palate, and tonsils

Clinical Clue Patients with herpangina often present to the pediatrician rather than the dentist, with a chief complaint of sore throat. The clinical presentation is similar to aphthous stomatitis except that the ulcers are limited to the soft palate and tonsillar pillars.

Hand-Foot-and-Mouth Disease

Hand-foot-and-mouth disease is a highly contagious, symptomatic, and self-limiting, viral infection. It most often affects infants and children younger than 5 years. It occasionally occurs in adolescents and adults. Children and parents (if not previously exposed) may be affected at the same time. Symptoms include fever, reduced appetite, sore throat, malaise, mouth sores, and skin rash. Most cases occur in the summer and fall. Typically it spreads via the fecal-oral route.

Clinical appearance: Skin lesions present as a rash of flat discolored spots and bumps which can be followed by vesicles or blisters. The rash is rarely itchy in children.

Oral lesions begin as red macules that evolve into 2–3 mm vesicles with an erythematous base which rapidly ulcerate. The ulcers are painful. The total number of oral lesions averages between 5 to 10. The tongue can also be edematous and tender.

Etiology: Coxsackie virus or Enterovirus. Coxsackie virus A16 is the most common cause followed by Enterovirus 71 (EV-71).

Location: Skin rash on palms of the hands, soles, buttocks, and sometimes around the nose or mouth. Oral lesions involve the palate, buccal mucosa, gingiva, and tongue.

Differential diagnosis: Aphthous stomatitis, erythema multiforme, various viral infections (i.e., herpangina, varicella-zoster, and primary herpes).

Treatment: Hand-foot-and-mouth disease is self-limiting, in which the rash and oral lesions resolve within 7–10 days. Treatment consists of supportive care—including maintaining fluid intake. Eating popsicles can also help soothe a sore throat. Topical anesthetics (i.e., viscous lidocaine) and/or a mouth rinse containing Benadryl and Kaopectate can be prescribed as a rinse and spit or can be applied directly to the lesions using a cotton swab in children over the age of three (see Medication Warning pg 36). OTC children's acetaminophen can also be helpful. If the child is immunocompromised or if the child is less than 6 months the patient's pediatrician should be notified.

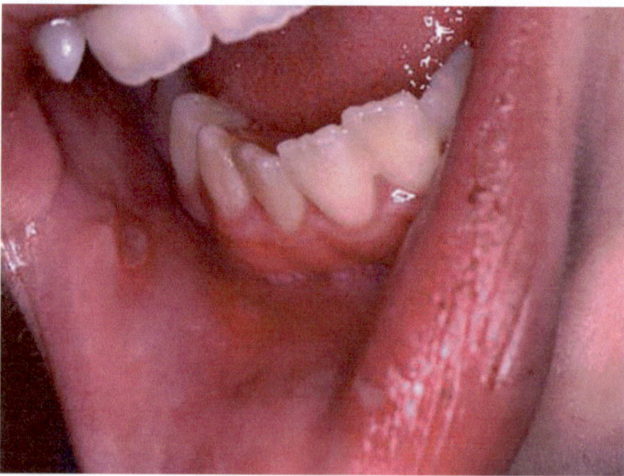

Fig. 1.57 Hand-foot-and-mouth disease. Aphthous-like ulcers with surrounding erythema involving the anterior buccal mucosa

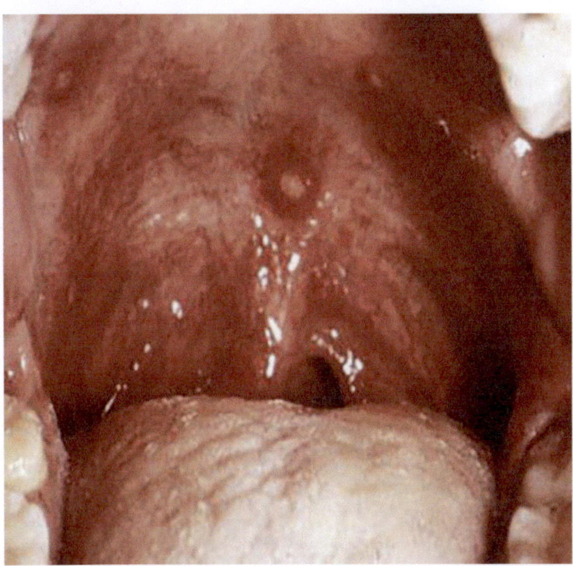

Fig. 1.58 Hand-foot-and-mouth disease. Punctate ulcers with surrounding erythema involving the soft palate. The patient presented with fever and sore throat

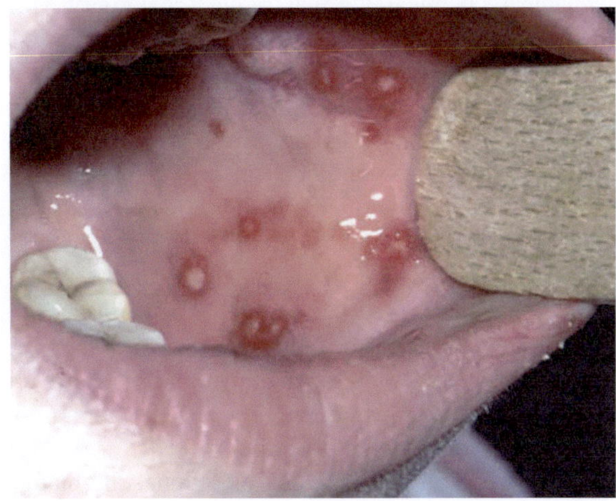

Fig. 1.59 Hand-foot-and-mouth disease. Multifocal aphthous-like ulcers with surrounding erythema involving the anterior buccal mucosa

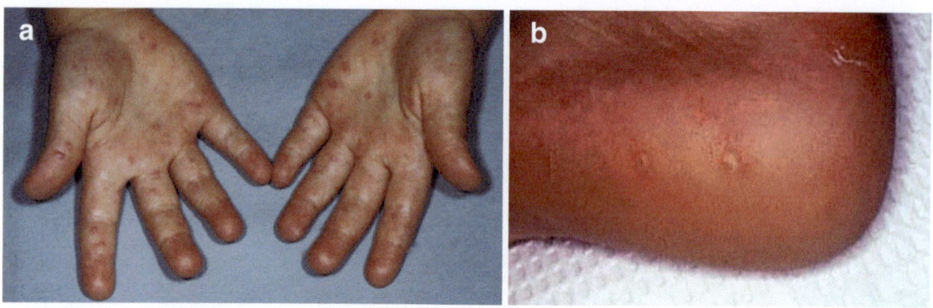

Fig. 1.60 (**a, b**) Hand-foot-and-mouth disease. Multiple small blisters and vesicles of the palms and soles

Clinical Clue Although the oral lesions are clinically non-specific, the characteristic rash of flat discolored spots and bumps which can develop into vesicles or blisters on the skin of palms and soles allows for the clinical diagnosis to be rendered.

Traumatic Ulcer

Clinical appearance: Area with loss of the surface epithelium appears red and can be painful. As the ulcer heals the periphery becomes white from hyperplasia of the regenerating epithelium.

Etiology: Mechanical, chemical, thermal, or electrical injury. Mechanical injury is the most common and includes accidentally biting while talking, sleeping, or eating. In children, post-anesthetic biting following dental procedures is common. Additionally, sharp incisal edges or cusps from teeth and the presence of natal or neonatal teeth can cause traumatic ulcerations (*Riga–Fede disease*). Infants and young children sometimes develop traumatic ulcers on the palate from sucking a pacifier or their fingers (thumb)—so-called *Bednar's aphthae*. Additionally, nervous habits or self-injurious behaviors such as fingernail scratching of the gingiva can result in oral ulcers. Severe ulcerations can be the result of self-mutilation in children with certain psychiatric disorders, developmental disabilities, or rare syndromes such as Lesch-Nyhan syndrome.

Location: Anywhere; the lower lip, buccal mucosa, and lateral tongue are common spots for mechanical trauma, whereas the palate is a common spot for thermal burns and the lip commissures for electrical injury.

Differential diagnosis: Viral ulcers, fungal infections, and malignancy must be ruled out.

Treatment: Traumatic ulcers heal within 2 weeks, following the removal of the source of the trauma. Children with nervous habits or behaviors may require psychological intervention. Dental interventions include occlusal guards and lip bumpers. In rare extreme cases, tooth/teeth extraction may be required to prevent self-mutilation.

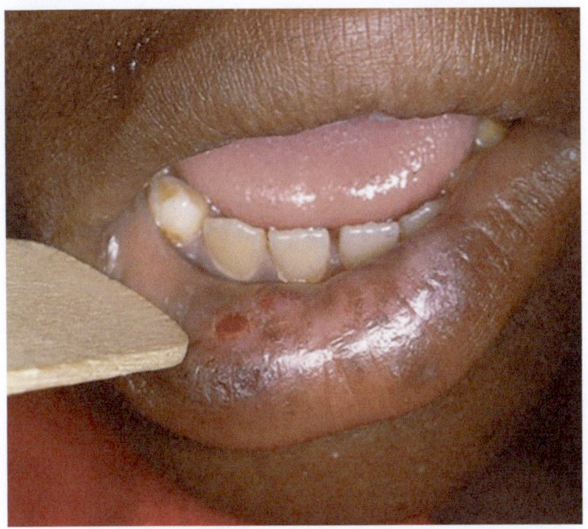

Fig. 1.61   Traumatic ulcer. Trauma from lower lip bite

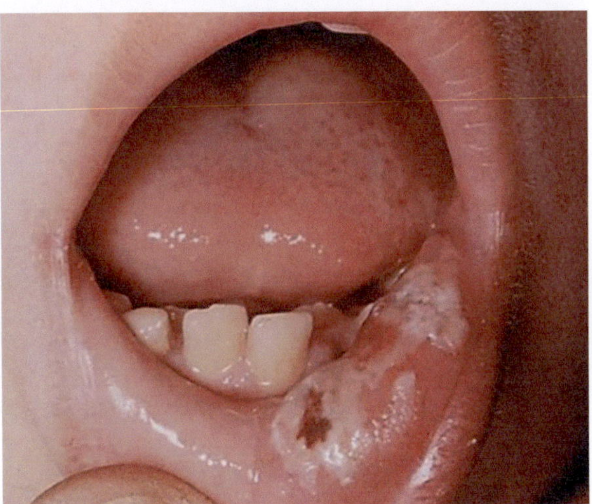

Fig. 1.62   Traumatic ulcer. Post-anesthetic lip bite

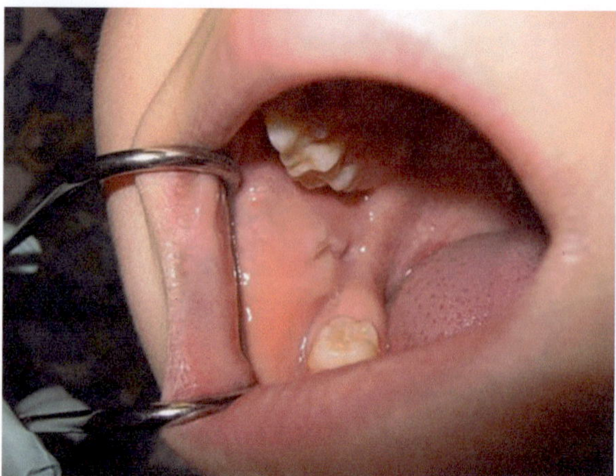

Fig. 1.63   Traumatic ulcer. Chronic linear ulceration of posterior buccal mucosa

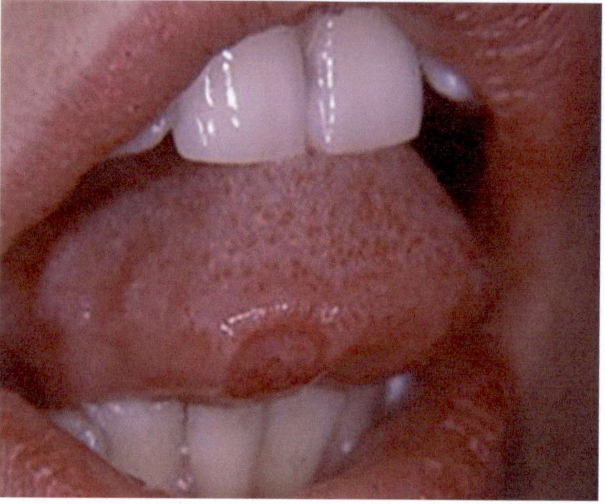

Fig. 1.64   Traumatic ulcer. Ulcer on the tip of the tongue, history of scalding

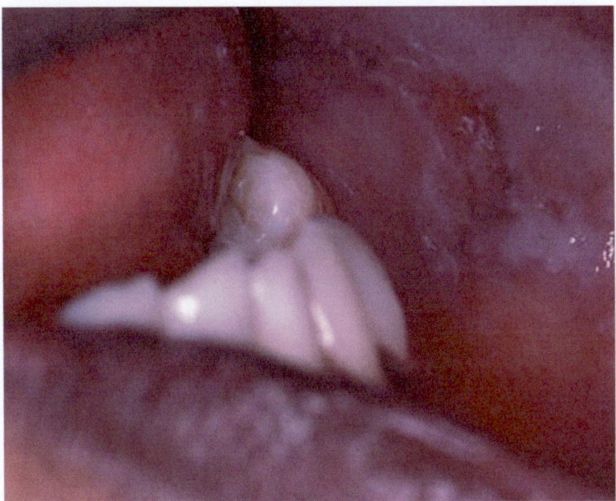

Fig. 1.65 Traumatic ulcer. Cheek bite, note the child also has leukoedema

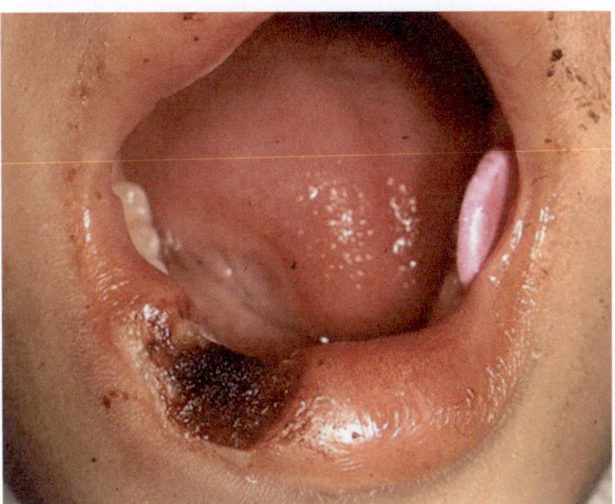

Fig. 1.66 Traumatic ulcer. Traumatic injury from an electrical burn

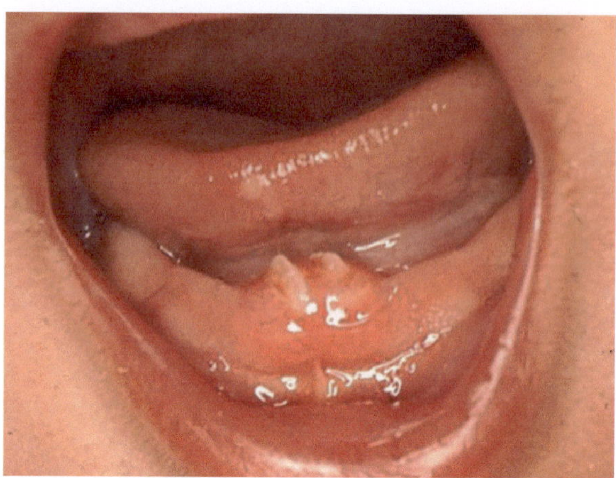

Fig. 1.67 Riga-Fede disease. Ulceration of the ventral tip of tongue an corresponding two erupting natal teeth

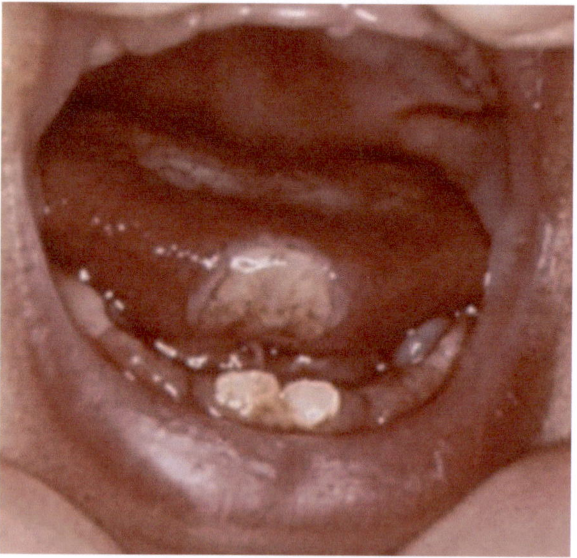

Fig. 1.68 Riga-Fede disease. Large ulceration of the ventral tip corresponding to natal teeth

Riga–Fede Disease
Ulceration of the ventral tongue or lower lip in newborns caused by trauma to the soft tissue from erupted natal teeth.

Clinical Clue Careful history-taking and examination are crucial in diagnosis of traumatic ulcers. Also, observing the patient for any habits can provide diagnostic clues. Trauma from an acute insult should heal within 2 weeks. However, if the patient repetitively or habitually traumatizes the site then the lesion(s) will persist and some form of intervention is required. If the lesion(s) persist despite intervention—biopsy is warranted. Self-induced or factitious injury should be kept in mind for unexplained oral mucosal lesions.

Recurrent Aphthous Stomatitis (aka canker sores or "Mikulicz aphthae)
The condition is characterized by round shallow periodic ulcers with a white or yellow center surrounded by red halo. Ulcers are painful, and depending on the location, it may be uncomfortable to eat or talk. There are three different types—minor, major, and herpetiform. A multifocal outbreak is referred to as aphthous stomatitis. Ulcers can occur periodically.

Recurrent aphthous stomatitis minor

Clinical appearance: The minor type is by far the most common. Minor aphthae are typically 2–4 mm in diameter and can occur as solitary or multiple (usually <6), each lasting 7–14 days.

Etiology: Not fully understood but thought to involve a T cell-mediated immune response triggered by a range of factors. Reported triggers/predisposing factors include nutritional deficiencies, local trauma (including orthodontic braces), stress, hormonal levels, allergies, and genetics.

Location: Minor aphthae occur *only on non-keratinized mucosa.*

Differential diagnosis: If focal—traumatic ulcer, if multiple—herpangina.

Treatment: Ulcers heal completely in 1–2 weeks and often do not require treatment. If the ulcers are such that they are interfering with the child's ability to eat or causing discomfort, topical corticosteroids, such as triamcinolone in Orabase®, can be used to lessen the pain. A topical numbing agent can also be used such as viscous lidocaine for children over three (see Medication Warning **pg 36**). For a multifocal outbreak, a short course of systemic prednisone can be beneficial. These medications must be used with supervision in children. For infants and young children, it is prudent to consult with the patient's pediatrician before prescribing corticosteroids.

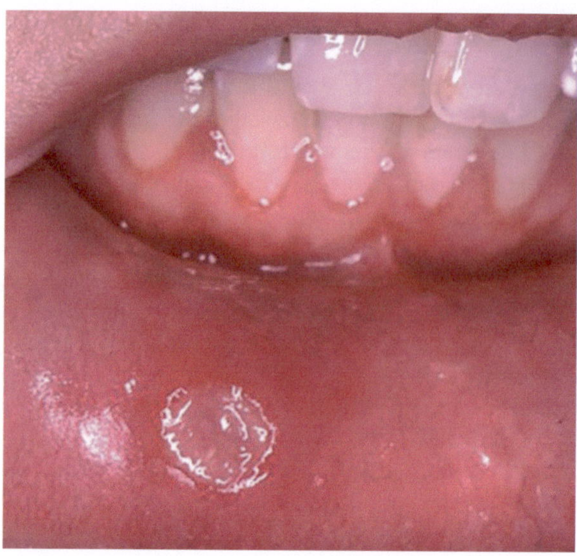

Fig. 1.69   Minor aphthous ulcer. Single round ulcer of the lower lip

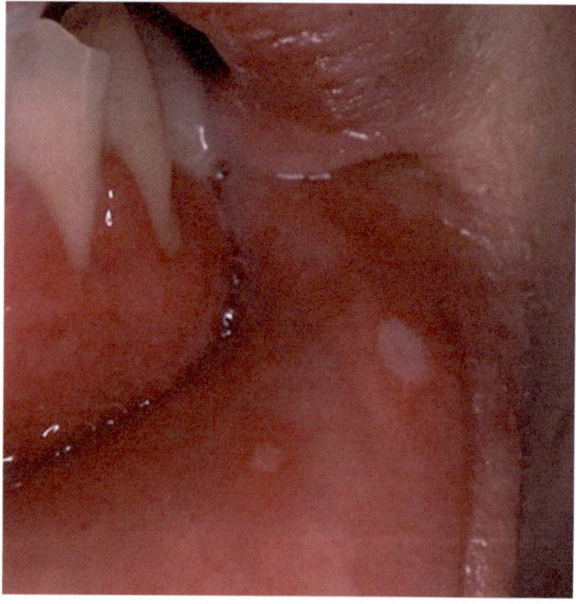

Fig. 1.70   Minor aphthae. Circumscribed ulcerations of the lower lip with faint erythematous halos

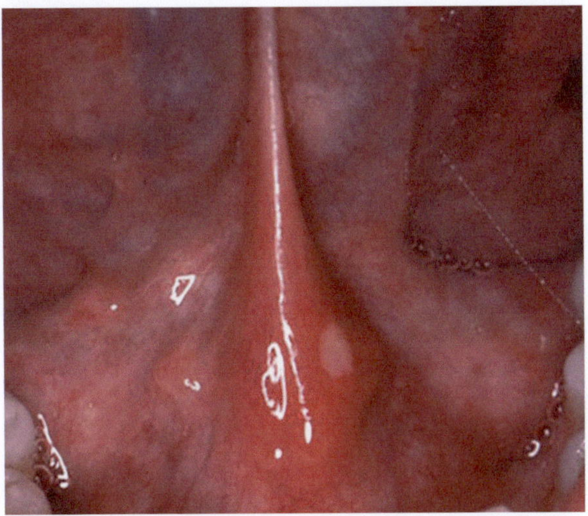

Fig. 1.71 Minor aphtha. Focal circumscribed tan-white ulcer with peripheral erythema involving the base of the lingual frenum

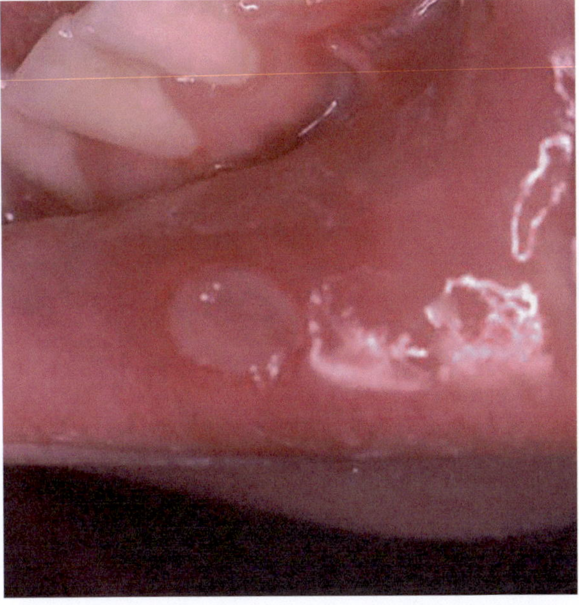

Fig. 1.72 Minor aphtha. Focal circumscribed tan-white ulcer of the lower lip with peripheral erythema

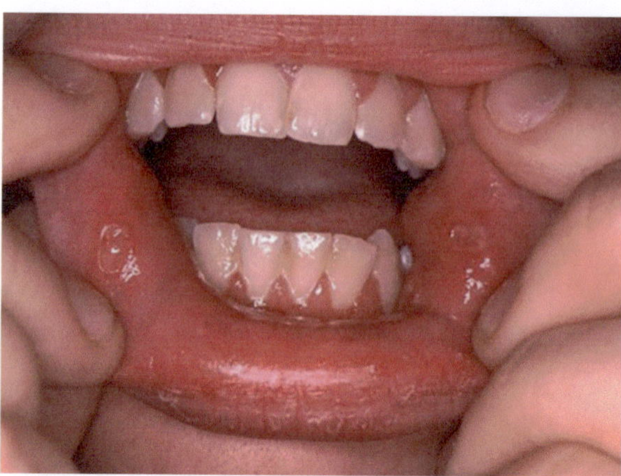

Fig. 1.73 Aphthous stomatitis minor. Two minor aphthae of the right and left lower lip/commissure areas

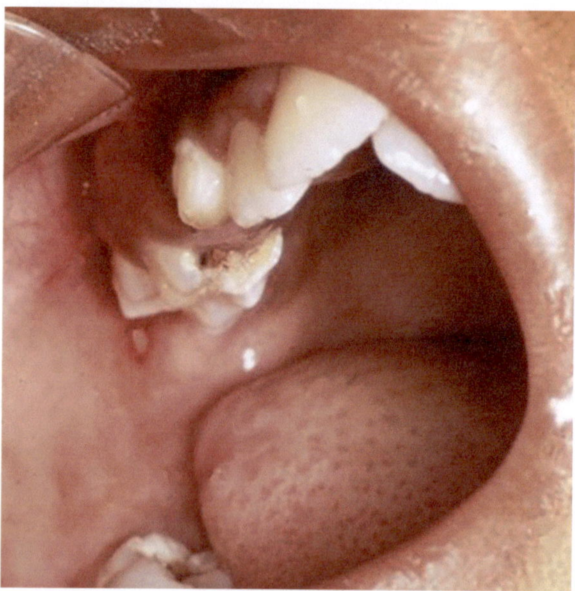

Fig. 1.74 Minor aphtha. Focal ulcer with erythematous halo of the posterior buccal mucosa

Clinical Clue Location of the lesion(s) can help discriminate between recurrent aphthous stomatitis minor and herpetic ulcers. Minor aphthae occur *only on non-keratinized mucosa*.

Recurrent Aphthous Stomatitis Major

Major aphthae are similar to minor aphthous ulcers, but are deeper and larger in size, often more than 10 mm in diameter, and might have a more irregularly shaped border. Healing also takes longer, up to 6 weeks, and the ulcer could leave a scar. Although, major aphthae most often occur on non-keratinized mucosa, occurrence on keratinized mucosa can be observed.

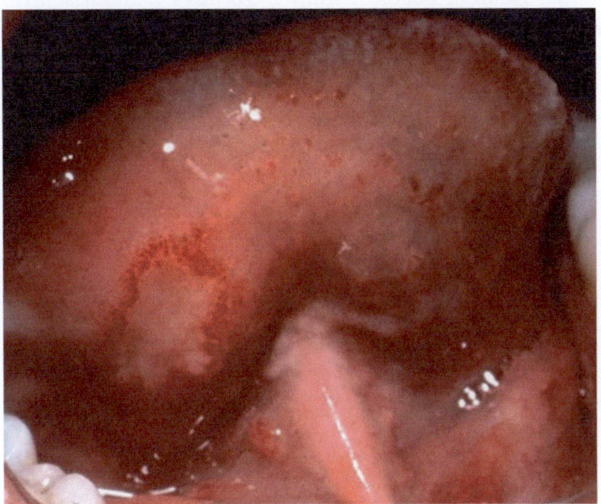

Fig. 1.75 Major aphtha. Large (>3 mm) tan-grayish irregular ulceration of the ventral tongue with surrounding erythema

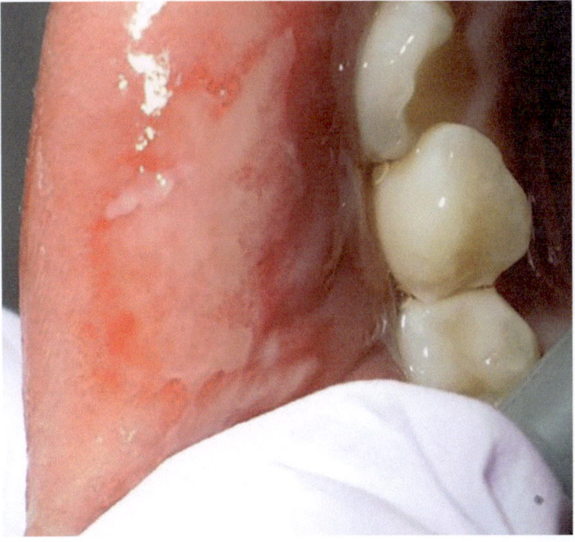

Fig. 1.76 Major aphtha. Large tan-grayish irregular ulceration involving the upper lip mucosa with an erythematous periphery

Recurrent Aphthous Stomatitis Herpetiformis

The lesions resemble a primary herpetic infection, thus the term herpetiformis. However, these ulcers are not caused by herpes virus and they are not preceded by vesicles, as is the case in a herpetic infection. The ulcers are smaller than those of minor aphthae, often less than 1 mm in diameter, and occur in clusters of up to 100 at a time. Adjacent ulcers merge to form larger, continuous areas of irregularly shaped ulcerations. Healing occurs within 7–10 days without scarring. Ulcerations can occur on either non-keratinized or keratinized mucosa. Herpetiform aphthae are often extremely painful, and the lesions recur more frequently than minor or major aphthae. Herpetiform aphthae typically occur in adolescents and young adults.

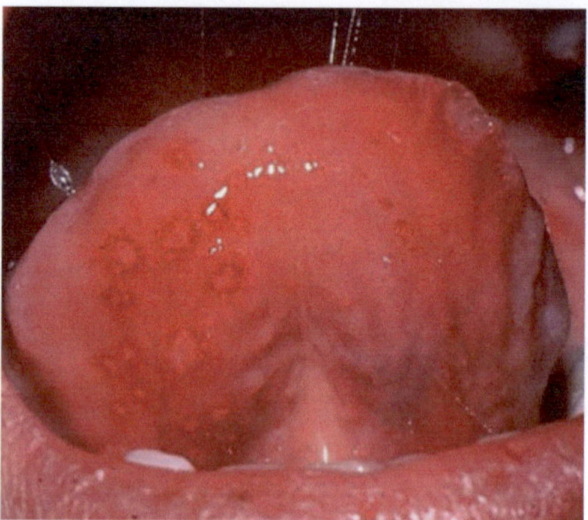

Fig. 1.77 Herpetiform aphthae. Numerous punctate ulcers of the ventral tongue

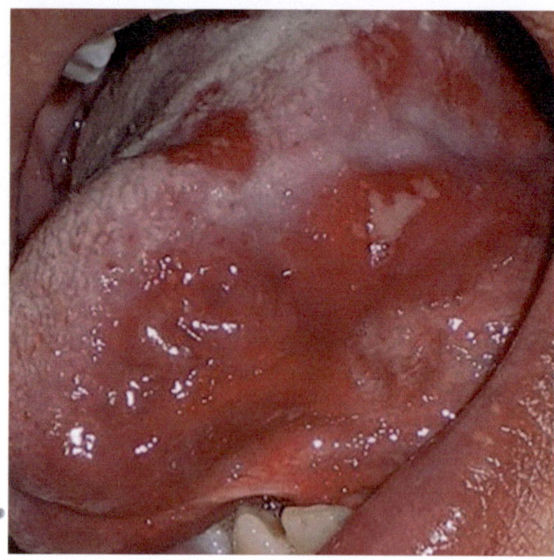

Fig. 1.78 Herpetiform aphthae. Punctate ulcers which have merged forming larger, irregular ulcerations

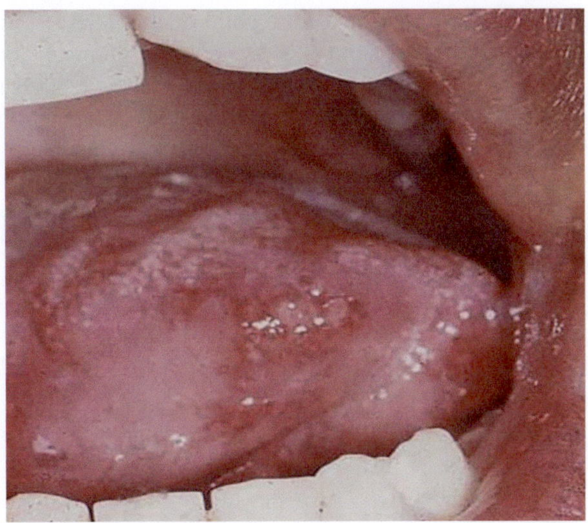

Fig. 1.79 Herpetiform aphthae. Punctate ulcers which have merged with larger, irregular ulcerations

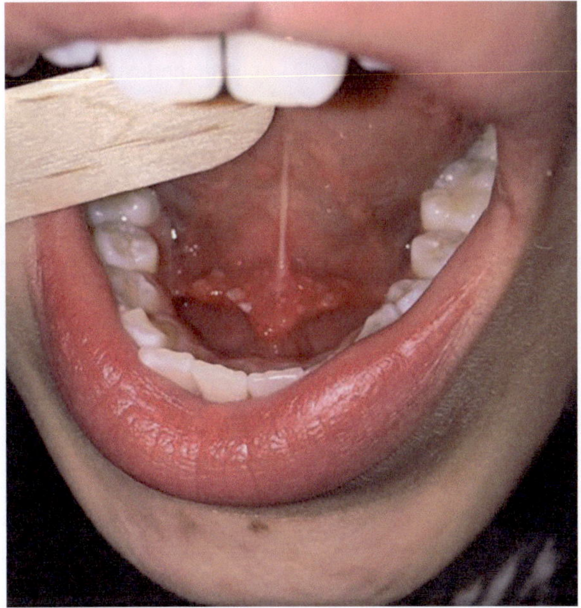

Fig. 1.80 Herpetiform aphthae. Numerous punctate ulcers of the floor of mouth

As mentioned, it is not uncommon for a child or an adolescent to get periodic outbreaks of recurrent aphthous stomatitis. However, if outbreaks occur consecutively, i.e., as soon as one ulcer heals another form and the patient is not without at least one ulcer at any given time, then it is important to investigate for an underlying systemic cause. Medical conditions that should be considered are listed in the table below.

Systemic conditions to consider as an underlying cause of Recurrent Aphthous Stomatitis in children and adolescents
Celiac disease
Inflammatory bowel disease
Cyclic neutropenia
Immunodeficiency/Immunosuppression
Nutritional deficiencies (iron, zinc, B vitamins)
Periodic Fever Aphthous stomatitis, Pharyngitis Adenitis (PFAPA) syndrome
IgA deficiency

Erythema Multiforme

Erythema multiforme (EM) is divided into minor and major forms. Lesions of EM minor are limited to the skin and one mucosal site (frequently the oral cavity). EM major involves the skin and at least two mucosal sites (i.e., conjunctiva, oral cavity, and genitourinary).

Clinical appearance: The presence of target-shape lesions on the skin is highly characteristic of EM. However, the clinical appearance of the skin lesions is variable. In addition, cases of erythema multiforme without cutaneous lesions have been recognized. Mucosal lesions, if present, typically develop a few days after the skin rash begins. The onset is abrupt.

Oral lesions begin as erythematous patches that undergo epithelial necrosis and evolve into large, shallow, irregularly shaped, and painful ulcers. Typically, the lips are swollen with hemorrhagic crust. The lesions are painful and the patient can have difficulty speaking or swallowing which can result in hospitalization often due to dehydration.

Etiology: EM is considered a type IV hypersensitivity reaction. Half of the cases are associated with certain infections (Mycoplasma pneumonia, HSV) or medications (antibiotics, e.g., sulfonamides, penicillin, and analgesics).

Recurrent episodes are often related to HSV infection.

Location: Ulcerations occur on both keratinized and non-keratinized mucosa. The tongue, buccal mucosa, and lips are most frequently involved. The gingiva and hard palate are relatively spared.

Differential diagnosis: Primary herpetic gingivostomatitis, mucosal pemphigoid, pemphigus vulgaris.

Treatment: EM is acute and self-limiting, usually resolving within 2–6 weeks. Topical numbing agents and pain medications can be used to ease discomfort and help the patient to maintain fluid intake and nutrition. The use of systemic steroids is controversial; however, it is the authors' experience that the oral lesions of EM respond rapidly to a short, tapered dose of oral steroids. In recurrent cases triggered by HSV, prophylaxis with oral acyclovir or valacyclovir can prevent recurrences.

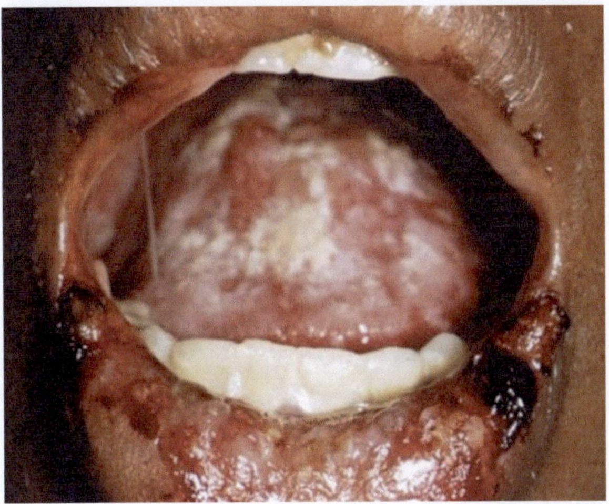

Fig. 1.81 Erythema multiforme. Bloody, crusted lips, characteristic of erythema multiforme, and oral ulcerations in a 12-year old

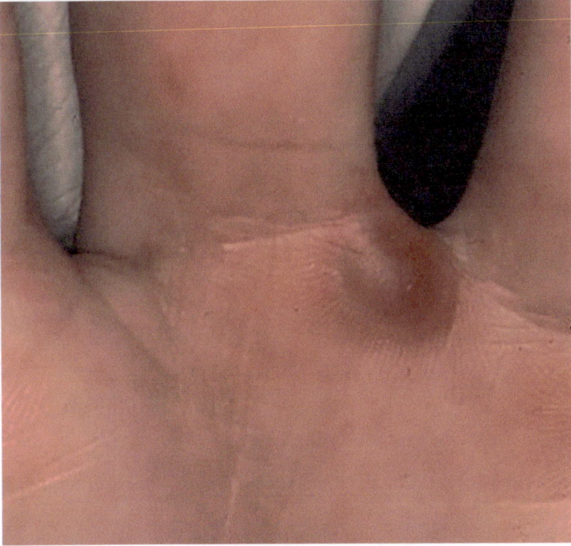

Fig. 1.82 Erythema multiforme. Targetoid cutaneous lesion in a child with erythema multiforme. The presence of targetoid skin lesions can help with the diagnosis, however, they are not present in every case

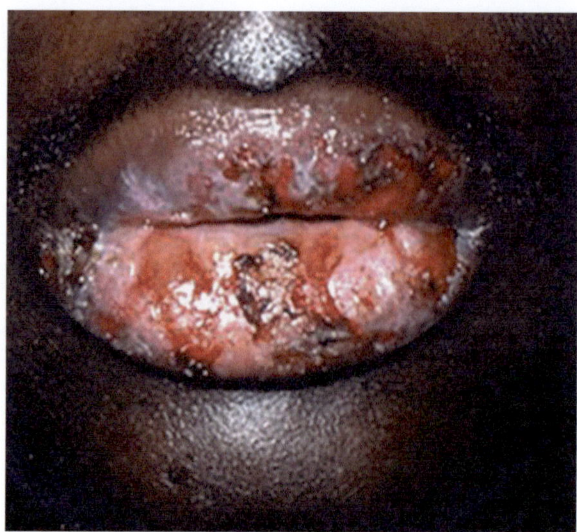

Fig. 1.83 Erythema multiforme. Ulcerated, crusted lips characteristic of erythema multiforme

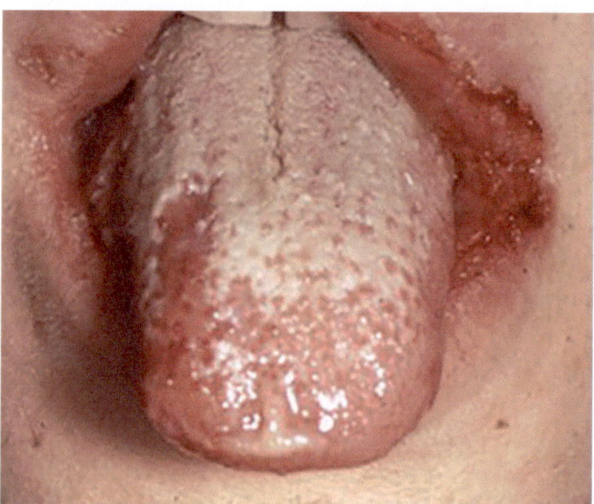

Fig. 1.84 Erythema multiforme. Bloody, crusted lips, and tongue ulcerations

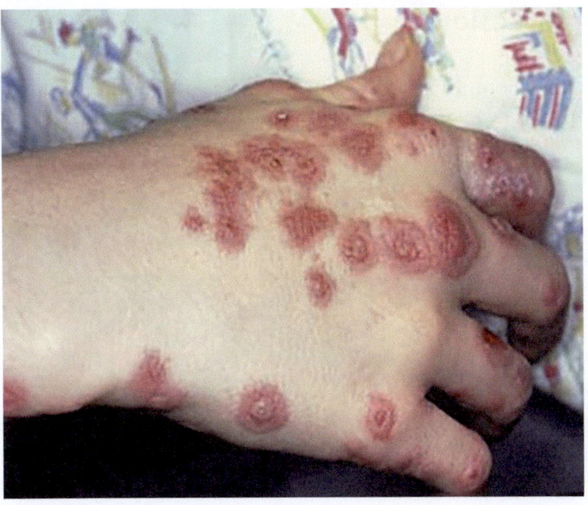

Fig. 1.85 Erythema multiforme. Cutaneous targetoid lesions of hand of the child shown

Clinical Clue Bloody, crusted lips with minimal gingival involvement can help to distinguish EM from primary herpetic gingival stomatitis. Also, patients can get recurrent bouts of EM whereas primary herpetic gingivostomatitis only occurs once. Pemphigus and pemphigoid are possible alternative diagnoses but they are much less common in children. Also, neither pemphigus nor pemphigoid is expected to be self-limiting.

Multifocal Oral Ulcers in a Child

Condition	Key features
Aphthous stomatitis	Often limited to non-keratinized mucosa
Acute Herpetic Gingivostomatitis	Gingiva is almost always involved, preceded/accompanied by fever, sore throat, malaise
Erythema multiforme	Bloody, crusted lips Possible preceding exposure to medications (antibiotics, analgesics)
Herpangina	Ulcers limited to soft palate and oropharynx
Vesiculobullous diseases (pemphigus, pemphigoid)	Rare in pediatric patients, lesions are not self-limiting, and tend to worsen until treatment is received
Hand, foot, and mouth disease	Common and highly contagious viral infection that causes painful ulcers in the oral cavity and throat. Characteristic, red spots or blisters on the hands, feet, buttocks, and thighs

1.3   Perioral Lesions

During dental treatment a variety of perioral lesions can be encountered. The entities below are likely to be encountered in pediatric patients.

Perioral Lesions
Herpes labialis
Impetigo
Perioral dermatitis
Lip lickers dermatitis

Herpes Labialis

Reactivation of the herpes simplex virus 1 (HSV-1) in a previously exposed child can result in intraoral (see Recurrent Intraoral Herpes pg 38) or extraoral lesions. The most common clinical form of recurrent infection is herpes labialis, commonly known as cold sore. Herpes labialis is often preceded by prodromal signs such as tingling or itching at the site and before development of clinical lesions.

Clinical appearance: Lesions consist of numerous tiny vesicles, which rupture rapidly to form ulcers. Cutaneous/labial ulcers become crusted.

Etiology: Herpes simplex virus 1 (HSV-1).

Location: Lip skin and vermillion.

Differential diagnosis: Impetigo, traumatic ulcer.

Treatment: Mild lesions typically heal without scarring in about a week, but healing can take up to 14–21 days for larger lesions. Prescription topical antiviral creams (i.e., Penciclovir 1% cream (Denavir)) or OTC topical antiviral cream Docosanol cream 10% (Abreva) can be helpful although they are most beneficial when applied at the earliest sign of an outbreak.

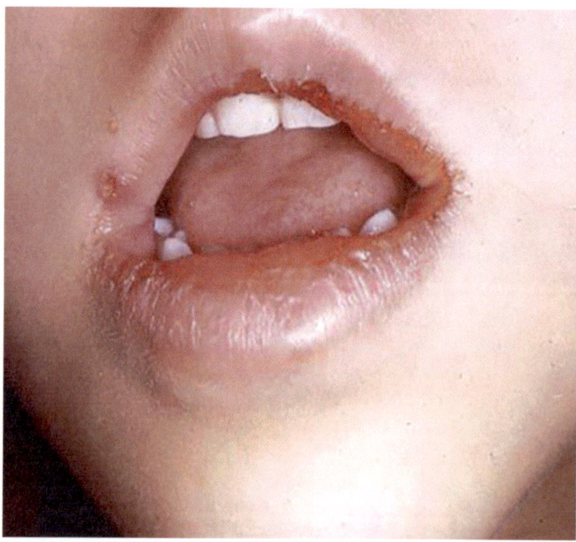

Fig. 1.86 Herpes labialis. Focal ulceration of the upper lip

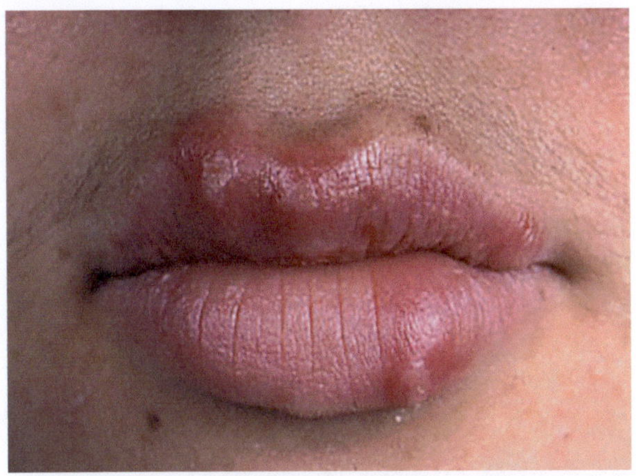

Fig. 1.87 Herpes labialis of the upper and lower lips

Reminder
Although the fluid-filled vesicles are the most infectious stage, all stages can be contagious.

Impetigo

Impetigo is a highly contagious *bacterial* skin infection common in children.

Clinical appearance: Multiple, scattered, discrete 1–3 cm cutaneous lesions with an *amber-colored crust* and surrounding erythema. There are several different types of impetigo. Impetigo contagiosa, also called non-bullous impetigo, is the most common type in children. The lesions might be itchy but are not painful.

Etiology: Staphylococcus aureus or Streptococcus pyogenes. Highly contagious.

Location: Facial skin around the mouth and/or nose. Often affects sites of trauma.

Differential diagnosis: Herpetic infection/Herpes labialis, candida infection.

Impetigo is usually diagnosed based on clinical appearance. Clinical diagnosis can be confirmed by performing a Gram stain or culture of the exudate from the lesion.

Treatment: Treatment options vary and range from washing with soap and water and letting the lesions air dry, to topical or oral antibiotics.

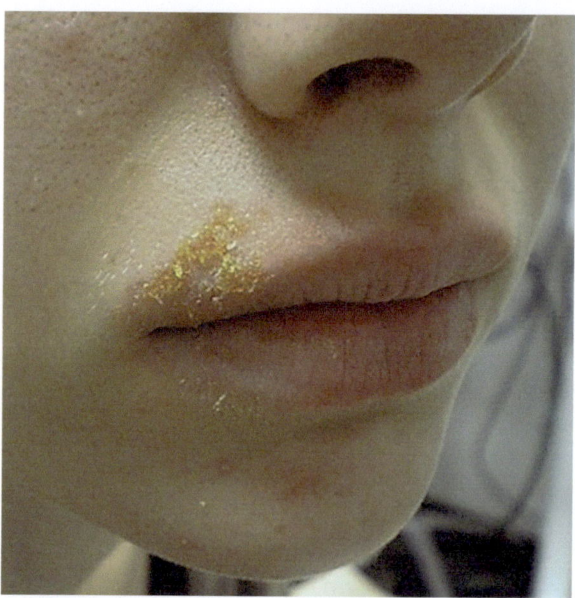

Fig. 1.88 Impetigo. Amber colored, corn flake-like crusting of skin of lip

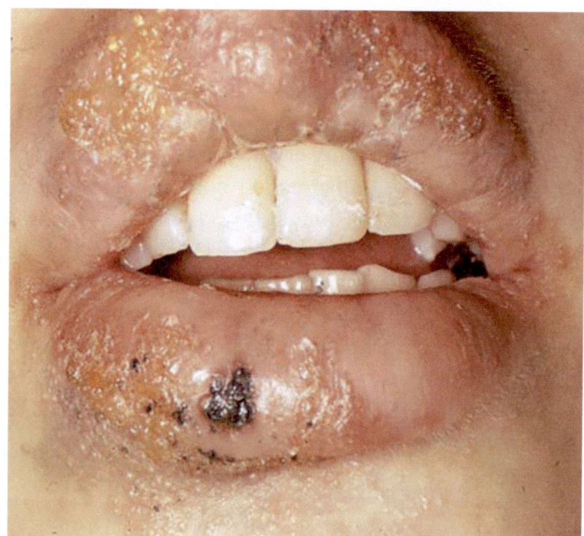

Fig. 1.89 Impetigo. Amber colored crusting of the upper and lower lips

Clinical Clue Duration of the lesion can help discriminate between herpes labialis and impetigo. Unlike herpes labialis which is expected to resolve without treatment in 7–10 days, impetigo can persist for longer if left untreated. Also, the crust in impetigo has a characteristic amber color and is sometimes described as having the appearance of "corn flakes."

Perioral Dermatitis

Perioral dermatitis is an acne-like eruption or rash commonly seen around the mouth in children and adolescents.

Clinical appearance: Multiple, small pink, acne-like bumps around the mouth and sometimes around the nose and eyes. The lesions do not involve the lips. The rash can be asymptomatic, mildly pruritic, or cause a burning sensation. The rash tends to wax and wane.

Etiology: The exact etiology is not known. The use of topical, inhaled, or nasal corticosteroids has been an established trigger in some cases. A theoretical cause is an overgrowth of normal skin mites and yeast. An irritant element is also believed to play a role in the development of perioral dermatitis. Examples of these irritants include moisturizers and other topical products applied to the face.

Location: Skin around the mouth and/or nose and eyes.

Differential diagnosis: Acne vulgaris, lip licker dermatitis, contact dermatitis.

Treatment: Treatment can be difficult and can involve multiple attempted modalities. Topical steroids can initially appear to help perioral dermatitis, however, the eruptions return and are more severe when the topical steroids are stopped. Despite the appearance that topical steroids are helping, it is important to discontinue the steroid application. The eruptions often take 3–6 weeks to fully improve.

The following management and treatment modalities have been reported to successfully clear perioral dermatitis:

- Remove triggers. As stated above, the use of topical steroids should be discontinued. If the patient uses an inhaled or nasal steroid, the patient should avoid having it in contact with their skin. Patients should also discontinue the application of any potentially irritating substances such as moisturizers.
- Topical antibiotics. Topical antibiotics such as clindamycin or erythromycin, are typically the next line of treatment for perioral dermatitis.
- Topical non-steroid anti-inflammatory creams. Topical non-steroid anti-inflammatory creams such as calcineurin inhibitors (i.e., tacrolimus ointment) can resolve the lesions in some patients.
- Anti-mite therapies. Anti-mite creams can be used to treat perioral dermatitis. Some patients have mild peeling after such use.
- Oral antibiotics. If the rash is severe or does not respond to topical creams, oral antibiotics have been reported to be successful in some patients. Older children are often treated with tetracyclines, whereas children under the age of 8 years are typically treated with azithromycin, erythromycin, and clarithromycin. This is because tetracycline can permanently stain the developing teeth.

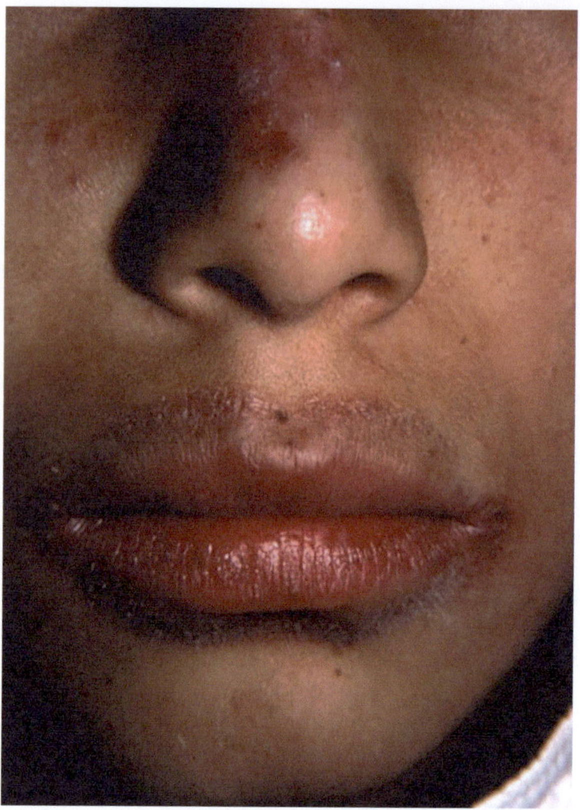

Fig. 1.90 Perioral dermatitis. Red and scaly rash encircling the mouth with involvement of skin of the nose

Lip Licker's Dermatitis

Lip licker's dermatitis (lip lick cheilitis, lip licking eczema) is a reaction of the lips and surrounding skin due to contact with saliva from chronic licking. Lip licker's dermatitis is most commonly seen in school-aged children, although it can present at any age.

Clinical appearance: Chronic redness, dryness, and scaling along the perimeter of the mouth. The skin can become cracked and inflamed leading to pain and itching.

Etiology: Excessive licking and wetting of the area surrounding the mouth is the direct cause of lip licker's dermatitis. The chronic wet-dry cycle of saliva from habitual licking upsets the normal skin barrier. This results in inflammation. The inflammation promotes further lip licking, continuing the cycle. Skin breakdown can lead to a secondary bacterial skin infection and/or fungal infection.

The licking can start as an attempt to relieve dry lips, as the condition is much more common in the winter, when children are more subject to dry lips and dry skin. Chronic lip licking can also become a subconscious habit in children that develops as a way to help manage anxiety, nervousness, or boredom.

Location: Lip and surrounding skin in a distribution that corresponds to the reach of the patient's tongue.

Differential diagnosis: Allergic contact cheilitis and allergic contact dermatitis, periorificial dermatitis.

Treatment: Discontinuation of lip licking is essential. Keeping the lips moisturized with a lip balm can help prevent dryness and thereby minimize the desire to lick the lips. Chronic lip licking, as a stress reducer or nervous action, might require behavior modification techniques and intervention from a psychology/psychotherapy expert. A topical steroid can help to reduce inflammation in significant cases. A topical antibacterial or antifungal medication might be needed for those cases that have become secondarily infected.

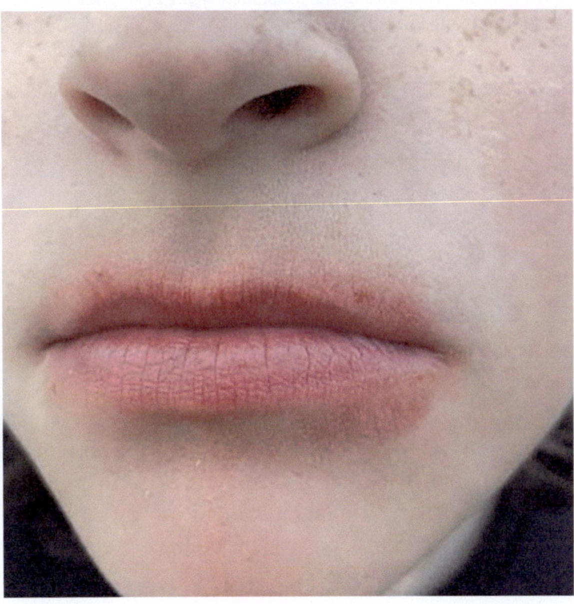

Fig. 1.91 Lip licker's dermatitis. Ten-year old with lip licking habit. Note the erythema and fine fissuring of lip vermillion and surrounding skin. The child complained of soreness and burning

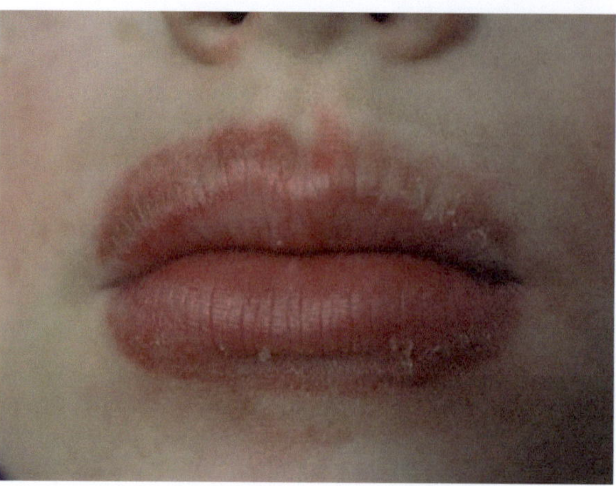

Fig. 1.92 Lip licker's dermatitis. The child presented with erythema, fine fissuring and focal exfoliation of lip vermillion and surrounding skin. *Photo courtesy of Dr. Andrea Mann*

Clinical Note

A distinguishing feature between perioral dermatitis and lip licker's dermatitis is that perioral dermatitis does not involve the vermilion of the lip or the skin immediately adjacent to the lip and generally causes papules.

1.4 White and Red Macules and Patches

It is not uncommon to encounter various white or red macules or patches in pediatric patients. These lesions are often transient and of various origins such as thermal insult, trauma, or frictional irritation. It is important to distinguish these lesions from true leukoplakias and erythroplakias, which are by definition premalignant lesions. Fortunately, true leuko- and erythroplakias are rare in children and adolescents.

White and Red Macules & Patches

Morsicatio Buccarum, Linguarum, and Labiorum
Superficial chemical burn
Oral Candidiasis
Allergic mucositis
Benign Migratory Glossitis
Leukoplakia
Erythroplakia

Morsicatio Buccarum, Linguarum, and Labiorum

Morsicatio buccarum and linguarum are also known, respectively, as chronic cheek, tongue, and lip biting/chewing.

Clinical appearance: The lesions are white lesions with thickened ragged surface. The involved area is often diffuse and lose superficial keratin fragments can sometimes be peeled off.

Etiology: Chronic conscious or subconscious habit of chewing on the cheek, tongue, or lip.

Location: Buccal mucosa, lateral tongue, or lip mucosa.

Differential diagnosis: Candidiasis, leukoplakia.

Treatment: The diagnosis is usually made on the clinical appearance. The lesions are harmless and no treatment is required. However, biopsy is recommended when etiology cannot be clinically confirmed.

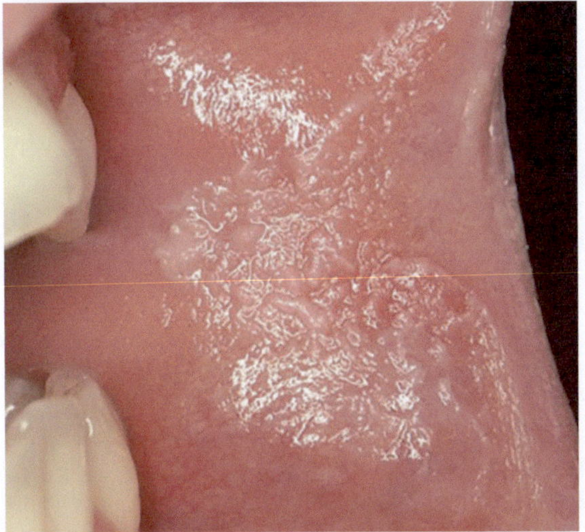

Fig. 1.93 Morsicatio buccarum. White ragged appearance of the anterior buccal mucosa in a teenager who chews on the area during studying

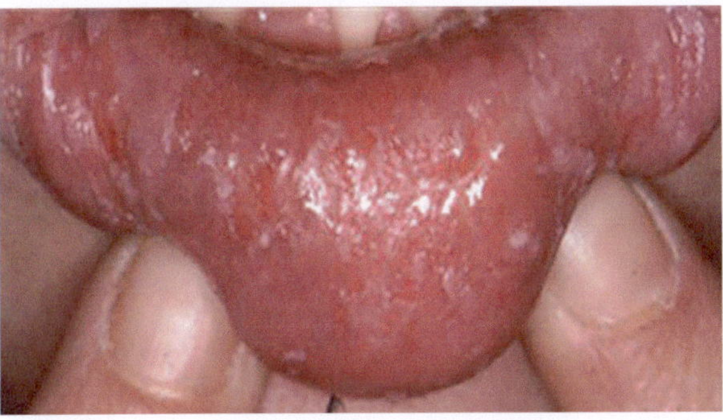

Fig. 1.94 Morsicatio linguarum. Ragged, macerated appearance of the lower lip. The patient has a lip chewing habit in addition to peeling off the loose "skin"

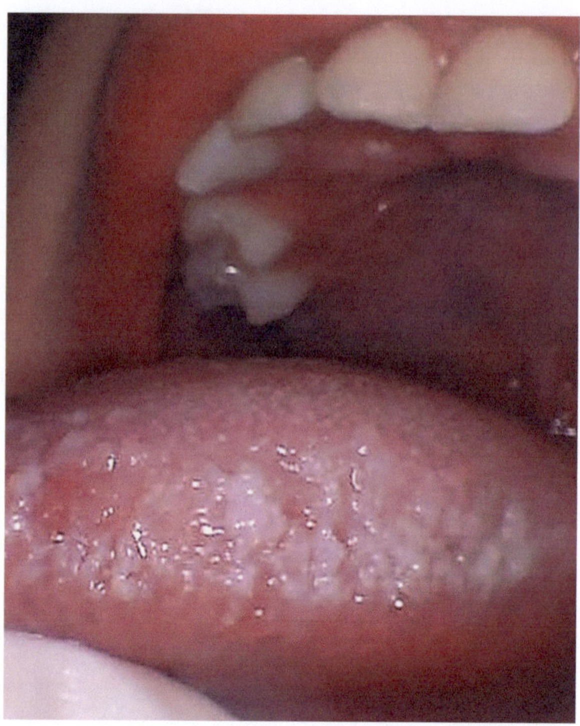

Fig. 1.95 Morsicatio linguarum. Irregular, white, and ragged appearance to the lateral tongue with focal intervening erythema in child with tongue chewing habit. *Photo courtesy of Dr. Andrea Mann, Basking Ridge, NJ*

Superficial Chemical Burn

Clinical appearance: Superficial sloughing or peeling of the mucosa. Patients often complain of wiping "stringy" material from their mouths in the morning.

Etiology: Superficial chemical burn often from dentifrice.

Location: Mandibular vestibule is the most common location.

Differential diagnosis: Mucous membrane pemphigoid, candidiasis.

Treatment: The diagnosis is based on the clinical finding of normal appearing mucosa beneath the superficially peeled off mucosa. This distinguishes it from vesiculo-erosive conditions such as mucosal pemphigoid. No treatment is required. The patient can switch to a mild toothpaste and avoid alcohol or peroxide-containing mouthwash.

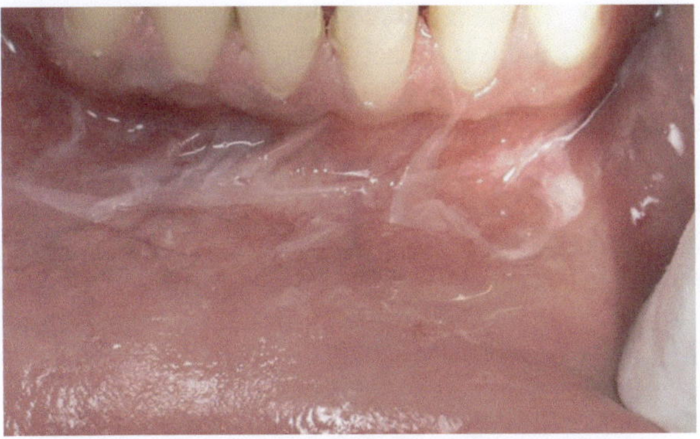

Fig. 1.96 Superficial chemical burn. Transparent white superficial sloughing of the mucosa. The sloughed mucosa is similar to a piece of thin wet tissue paper. Note the lack of any underlying erythema or erosion

Clinical Clue The superficial slough is transparent white and can be easily wiped off with a cotton-tipped applicator. The mucosa underlying the sloughed tissue is normal and asymptomatic.

Allergic Contact Stomatitis

Clinical appearance: Allergic contact stomatitis is a contact allergic reaction. Clinical presentation is variable. Lesions can present as erythema, edema, vesicles, erosions, and ulcerations. Some lesions can appear white or lichenoid.

Etiology: Common culprits include oral flavorings, preservatives, and dental materials. Cinnamon, particularly products containing cinnamon oil, are a common cause. Some examples seen in pediatric patients can be reactions to toothpaste, candy, and chewing gum (particularly those that are cinnamon flavored), acrylic monomer in orthodontic appliances and metal wires and topical anesthetics. Although counterintuitive, topical corticosteroids have also been implicated.

Location: Lesions of contact allergies occur adjacent to the area of contact with the triggering agent. The most common sites involved in contact stomatitis are the sides of the tongue, gingiva, buccal mucosa, and hard palate.

Differential diagnosis: The differential is dependent on the clinical appearance, which as stated is variable. Careful history-taking and clinical examination can help establish a cause-and-effect relationship.

Treatment: Once the potential trigger has been identified that agent should be removed, and the patient followed-up. Once the trigger is removed, the lesions should resolve in 1–2 weeks. Re-introduction of the offending agent can be a confirmatory test but is often not warranted.

Cinnamon contact stomatitis is a mucosal reaction to products containing artificial cinnamon flavor such as gum, hard candy, toothpastes, and mouthwashes. It manifests as red or thickened white mucosal patches in direct contact with the cinnamon flavored product. When associated with gum or candies, the lateral tongue and buccal mucosa are common sites. One side of the mouth, the side the child preferentially chews on or dissolves the candy against, is typically more affected than the contralateral side. The clinical diagnosis is confirmed by having the child discontinue the artificial cinnamon exposure.

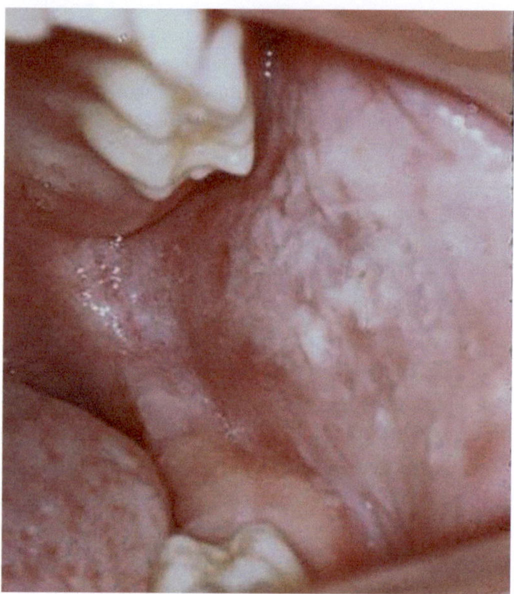

Fig. 1.97 Contact/Cinnamon Stomatitis. Diffuse white, focally thickened patch of the buccal mucosa

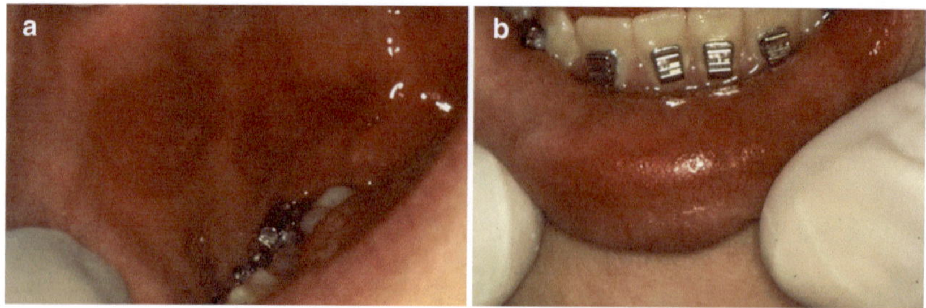

Fig. 1.98 (**a, b**) Contact Stomatitis. Reaction to orthodontic wire manifesting as painful, red patches of the buccal, and labial mucosa. Removal of the wire resulted in resolution within 4 days. *Photos 1.97 a & b appeared in Dunlap CL, Vincent SK, Barker BF. Allergic reaction to orthodontic wire: report of case, *The Journal of the American Dental Association*, 1989;118(4):449-450

Oral Candidiasis

Clinical appearance: Oral candidiasis can occur in three different clinical variants: Pseudomembranous (commonly referred to as thrush), erythematous or hyperplastic. The pseudomembranous form is the most common and presents as white removable plaques. Erythematous candidiasis presents with generalized erythema of the oral mucosa and the child might complain of a sore mouth. Hyperplastic candidiasis presents as white adherent plaques. Hyperplastic candidiasis is not commonly seen in children.

Etiology: Opportunistic fungal infection caused mostly by *Candida albicans*. It is important to note that since it is an opportunistic infection, a predisposing factor should be identified.

Location: Anywhere in the oral cavity; tongue, palate, and vestibules are common locations.

Differential diagnosis: Pseudomembranous candidiasis is not often confused with other entities since it is white to cream in color and wipeable. Erythematous candidiasis could be mistaken for geographic tongue, contact stomatitis, or allergy. Hyperplastic candidiasis might be mistaken for leukoplakia or geographic tongue. If a clinical diagnosis of oral candidiasis cannot be rendered, fungal culture, or cytologic smear or biopsy can be performed.

Treatment: Depends on age and severity.

- In infants younger than 6 months, thrush is fairly common and typically clears up on its own once the infant's immune system is fully established.
- In babies older than 9 months and in children, thrush is less common and an underlying cause should be sought. Nystatin oral suspension can be prescribed if the child is old enough to swish and spit. If the child is not capable of swish and spit, Nystatin oral suspension can still be prescribed with an instruction to the parents to "paint" the white patches with a sponge tip applicator or gauze-covered finger.

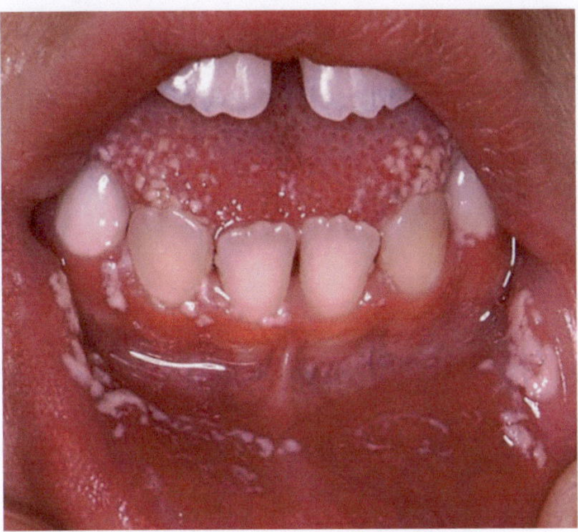

Fig. 1.99 Oral candidiasis, pseudomembranous type. Multiple white plaques of the lower labial mucosa, gingiva, and tongue. The associated mucosa is erythematous

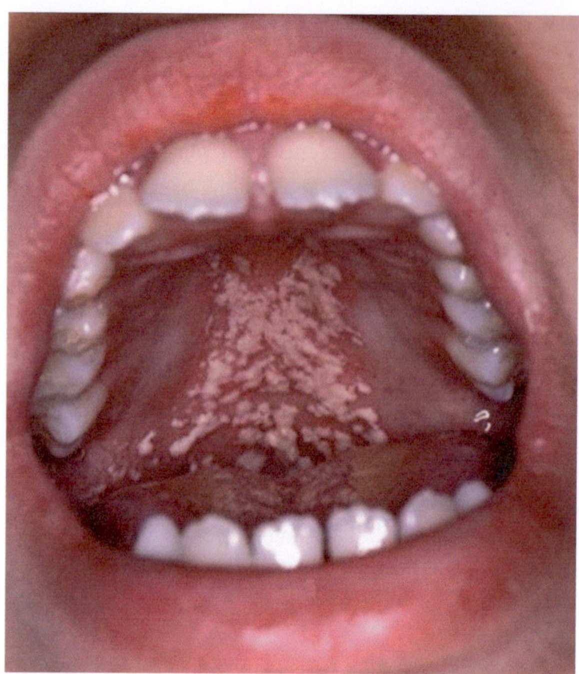

Fig. 1.100 Oral candidiasis, pseudomembranous type. Multiple white plaques of hard and soft palate

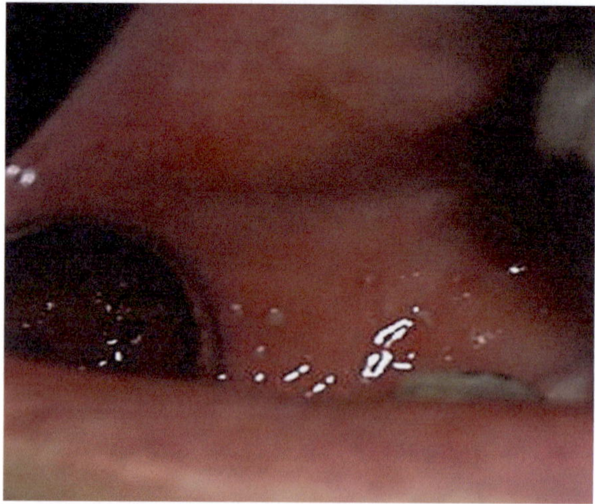

Fig. 1.101 Oral candidiasis, pseudomembranous type. Focal white plaques of buccal mucosa

Median Rhomboid Glossitis (central papillary atrophy) is considered a form of chronic candidiasis. It is characterized by an area of redness with loss of lingual papillae located on the midline of tongue dorsum. It is usually asymptomatic and treated with topical or systemic antifungal medication. Usually, the lesion disappears following the treatment although in some cases the resolution is incomplete.

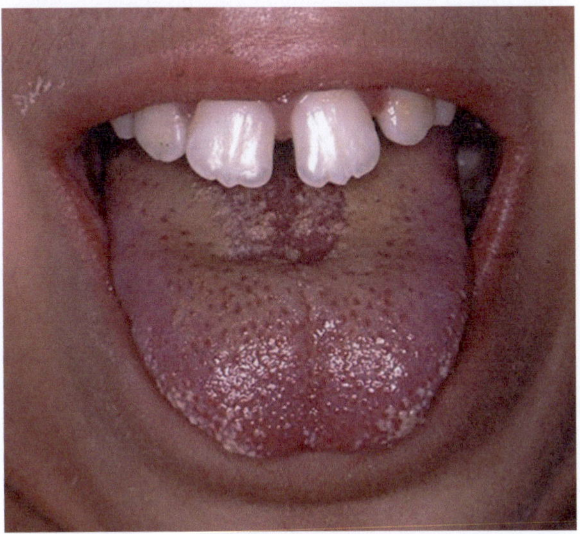

Fig. 1.102 Median Rhomboid Glossitis. Erythema and loss of papillae on the tongue dorsum midline

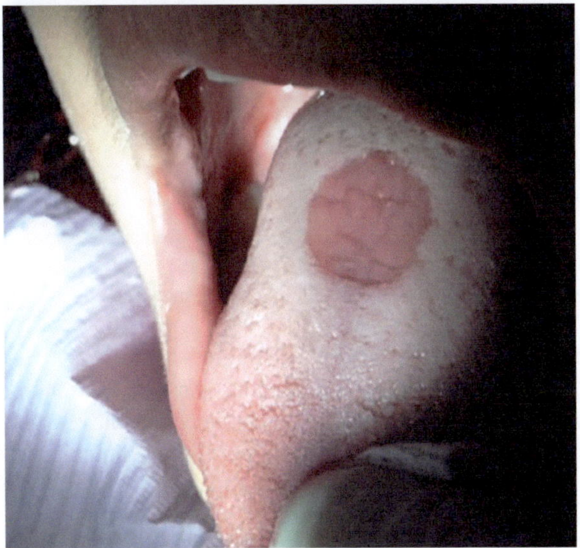

Fig. 1.103 Median Rhomboid Glossitis. Circular loss of lingual papillae on the tongue dorsum midline

Angular cheilitis is inflammation of one or both corners of the mouth. Often represents an opportunistic fungal and/or bacterial infection. Risk factors include nutritional deficiencies, decreased vertical dimension of the mouth, a lip licking habit, drooling, and immunosuppression. Although much more common in the elderly, it can also occur in children. The treatment is the application of antifungal, and/or antibacterial ointments with or without addition of a topical glucocorticoid steroid.

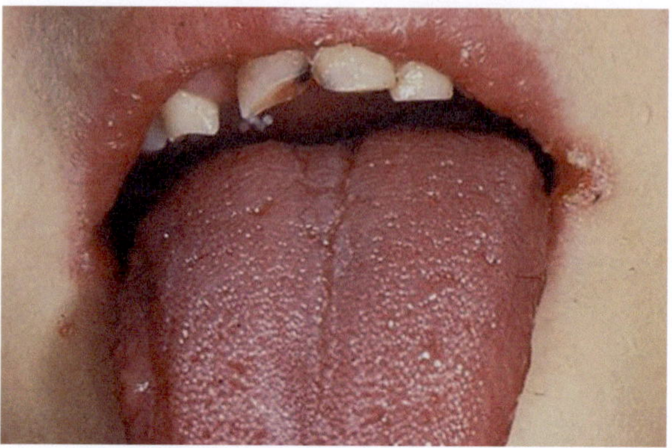

Fig. 1.104 Angular cheilitis. Erythema and cracking at the oral commissures

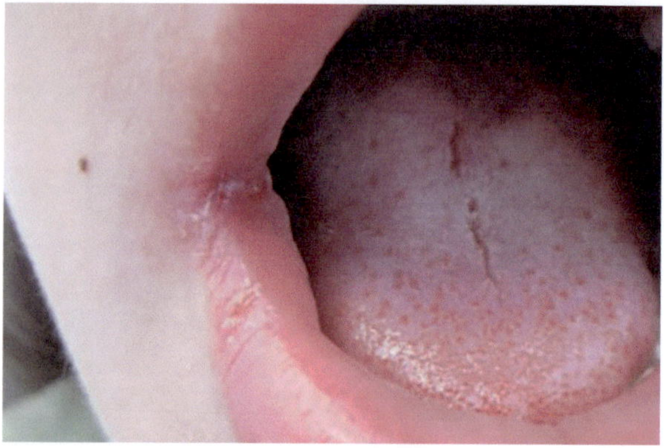

Fig. 1.105 Angular cheilitis. Fissure present in lip commissure

Benign Migratory Glossitis/Geographic Tongue

Geographic tongue, although common in adults, is not often seen in children.

Clinical appearance: Smooth, red, depapillated patches with a surrounding white serpentine border. The patches migrate over time. Clinical appearance is often diagnostic.

Etiology: Unknown, tends to run in families.

Location: Dorsum of tongue, can extend to lateral borders and infrequently affect other parts of the mouth (migratory stomatitis). In cases of the latter, the tongue is invariably involved.

Differential diagnosis: Can be misinterpreted as candidiasis, erythroleukoplakia, or lichen planus (the latter two rare in children).

Treatment: Treatment is not necessary. Rarely, some patients complain of a burning sensation and sensitivity to spicy foods, which is usually not a problem for children.

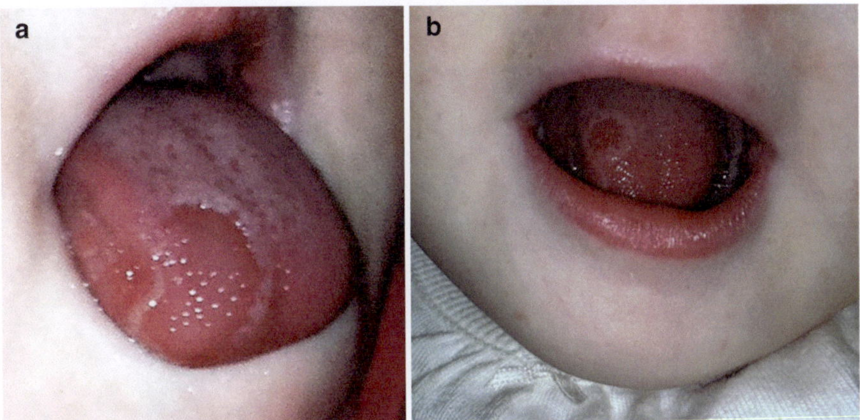

Fig. 1.106 (**a**, **b**) Benign migratory glossitis (geographic tongue). (**a**). Six-month-old with partially depapillated patches and surrounding serpentine border on the tongue dorsum. (**b**). After 5 days lesions have changed in shape and size

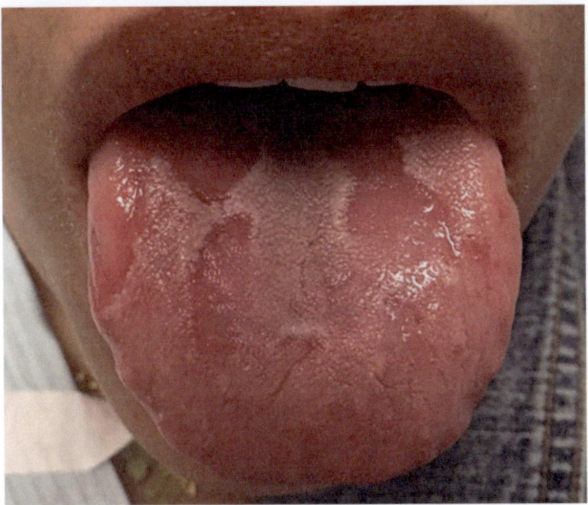

Fig. 1.107 Benign migratory glossitis. 16-year-old with smooth, depapillated patches with serpentine-like borders of the dorsal tongue extending to the lateral surface

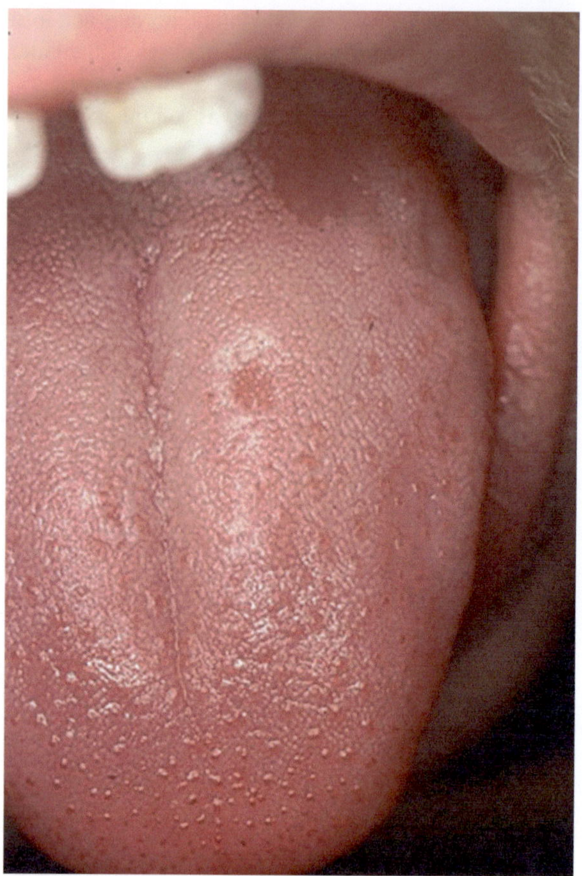

Fig. 1.108 Benign migratory glossitis. Subtle benign migratory glossitis

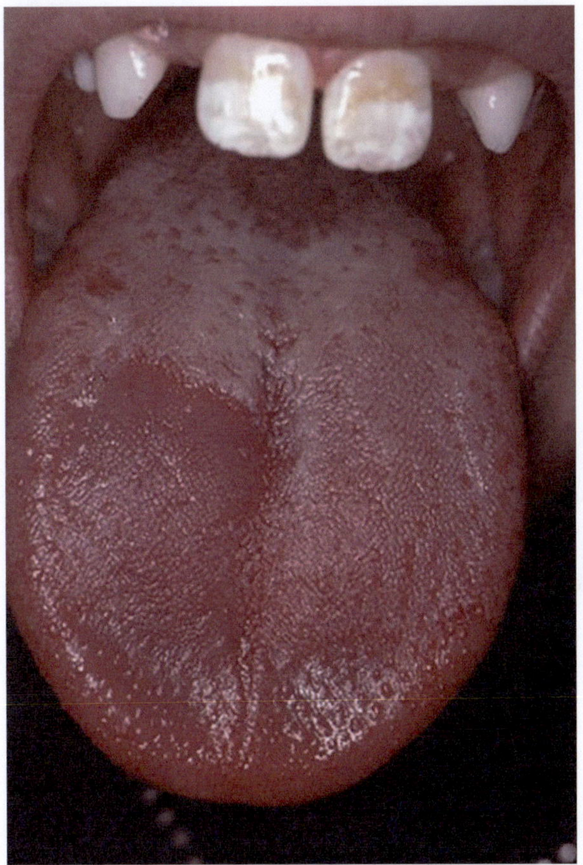

Fig. 1.109 Benign migratory glossitis. 8-year-old with depapillated patches of the dorsal tongue

Leukoplakia

Leukoplakia is a non-removable white lesion that cannot be characterized clinically or pathologically as any other disease. True leukoplakias are considered premalignant and are very rare in children.

Clinical appearance: A non-removable white or gray patch or plaque.

Etiology: Unknown.

Location: Any mucosal surface. The lateral tongue and floor of the mouth are high-risk areas.

Differential diagnosis: Morsicatio buccurum, morsicatio linguarum, candidiasis, geographic tongue, leukoedema, trauma, contact stomatitis.

Treatment: If the cause of the white lesion cannot be identified, or if it persists even after removing the source of irritation, biopsy is recommended.

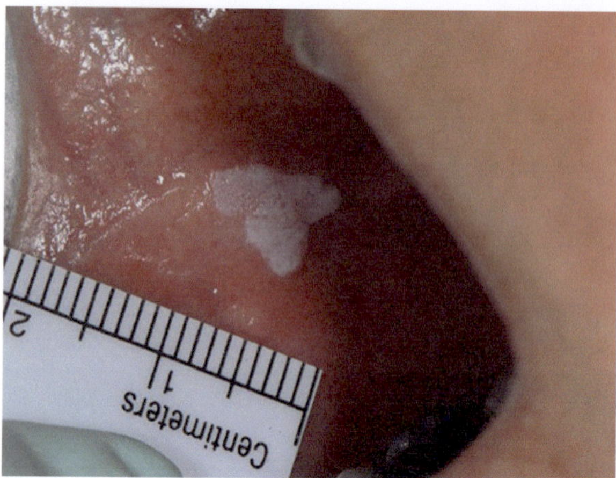

Fig. 1.110 Leukoplakia. Well demarcated leukoplakia of the buccal mucosa. No etiology was identified

Examples of "white" lesions that are *not* true leukoplakias.

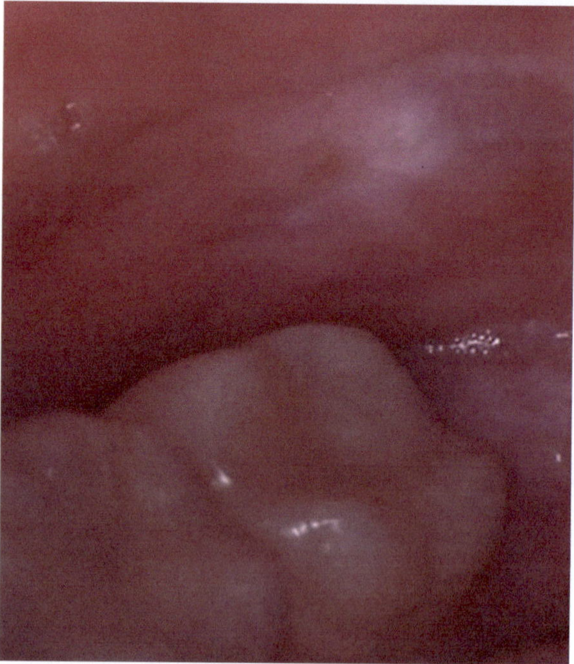

Fig. 1.111 Frictional keratosis. A white lesion that resulted from occlusal trauma. Posterior ridge keratosis can also be seen. Frictional keratosis is not considered a true leukoplakia

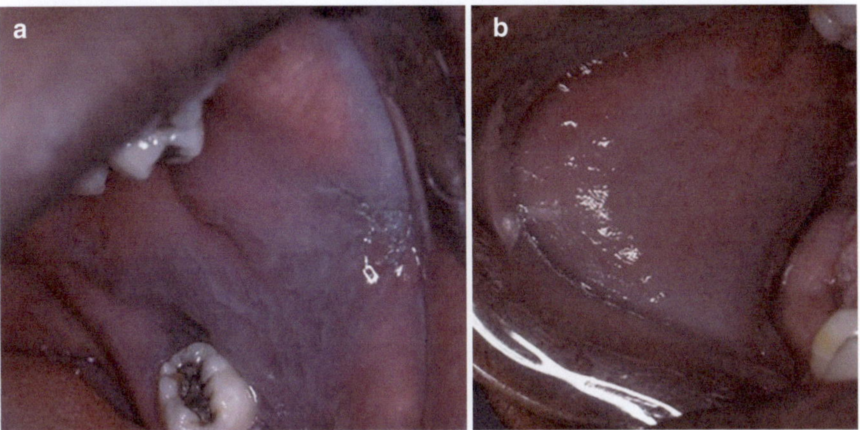

Fig. 1.112 (**a**, **b**) Leukoedema. White opalescent quality to bilateral buccal mucosa which disappears when the cheek is stretched (**b**). Leukoedema is considered a variation of normal and is not a leukoplakia

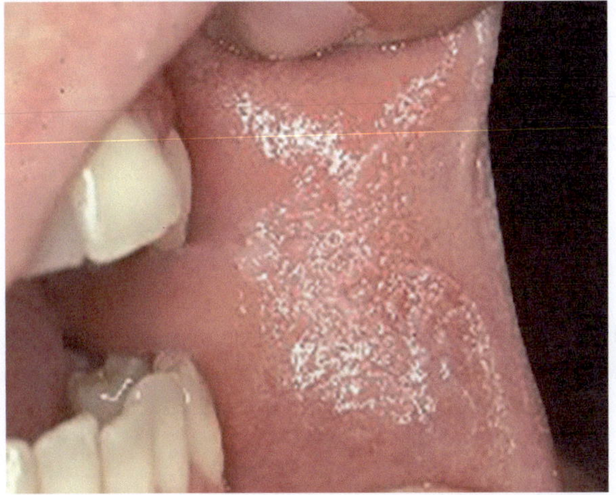

Fig. 1.113 Morsicatio buccarum. Irregular, white, and ragged appearance to the anterior buccal mucosa with faint intervening erythema in teenage patient with habit if cheek chewing

Erythroplakia

Erythroplakia is a red patch that cannot be characterized clinically or pathologically as any other disease. Erythroplakias are histologically severe dysplasias or squamous cell carcinoma at biopsy. Erythroplakias are very rare in children. They are included in this atlas because they can be confused with other more common red lesions.

Clinical appearance: A red patch with a smooth or granular surface, can have a mixture of red and white (erythroleukoplakia).

Etiology: Unknown, apparently similar to the causes of squamous cell carcinoma.

Location: Anywhere; high-risk sites include ventral and lateral tongue, floor of mouth, and soft palate/oropharynx.

Differential diagnosis: Erythematous candidiasis, geographic tongue, contact stomatitis, localized inflammation, trauma, vascular lesions.

Treatment: A red patch of the oral mucosa in a child is much more likely to be a lesion that mimics erythroplakia than true erythroplakia. That being said, if a red patch with uncertain etiology persists, a biopsy is required.

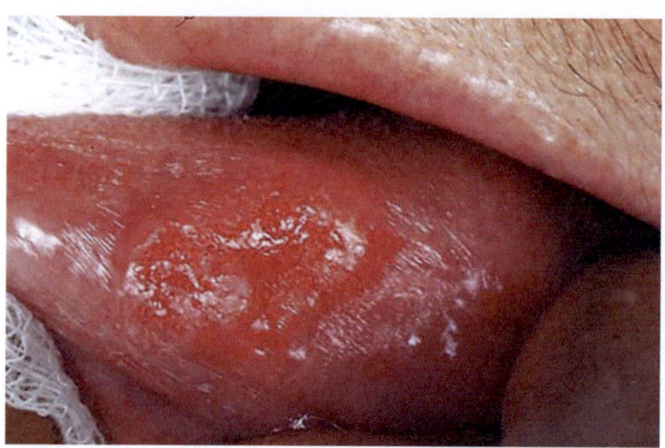

Fig. 1.114 Erythroplakia. Red patch of the lateral tongue in an adult patient. The lesion was asymptomatic

1.5　Gingival Lesions

In this section, focal and generalized gingival enlargements and gingivitis are discussed. When evaluating a gingival enlargement or nodule, it is prudent to take a radiograph of the area to ensure that the lesion is limited to the soft tissue.

Gingival Lesions
Pyogenic Granuloma
Peripheral Ossifying Fibroma
Fibroma/Giant Cell Fibroma
Peripheral Giant Cell Granuloma
Parulis
Eruption Cyst
Gingival/Alveolar Cysts of the Newborn
Localized juvenile spongiotic gingival hyperplasia
Gingivitis and generalized gingival enlargements

Pyogenic Granuloma

See page 16—for entity details. Clinical photographs of pyogenic granuloma of the gingiva are provided in Fig. 1.115–1.118.

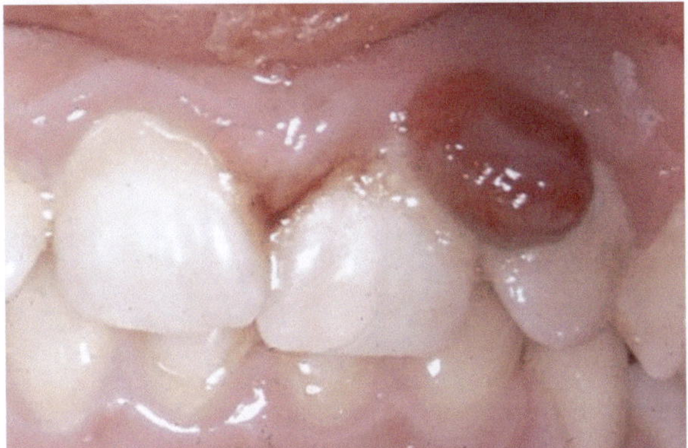

Fig. 1.115 Pyogenic granuloma. Erythematous exophytic nodule of the maxillary attached gingiva. Note the adjacent plaque accumulation

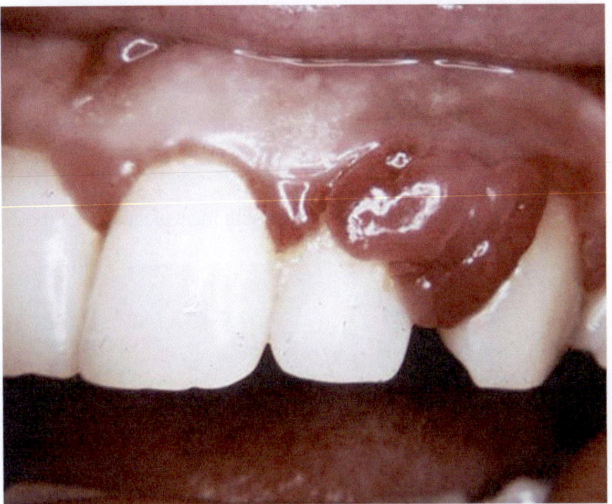

Fig. 1.116 Pyogenic granuloma. Erythematous nodule of the maxillary gingiva

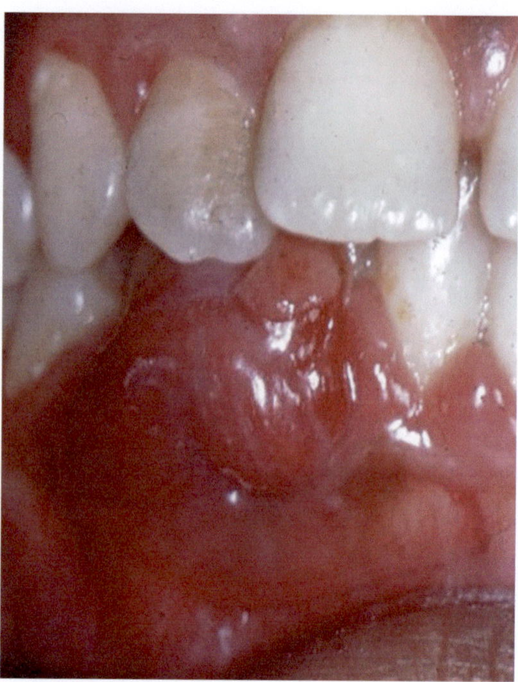

Fig. 1.117 Pyogenic granuloma. Erythematous growth with focal ulceration of the mandibular gingiva

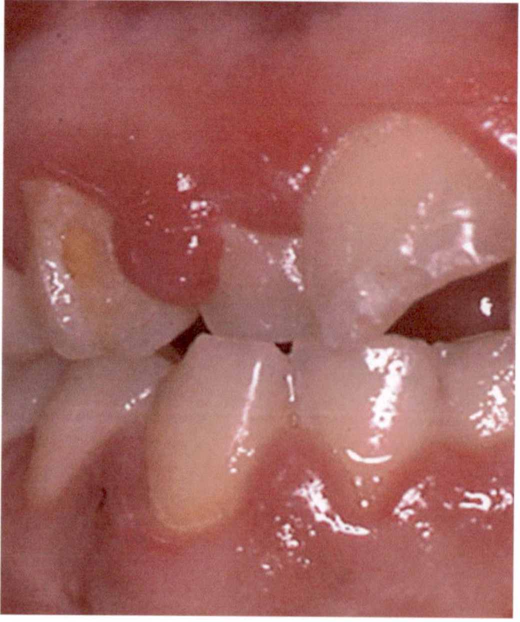

Fig. 1.118 Pyogenic granuloma. Erythematous nodule of the maxillary gingiva

Fibroma

See page 14 for entity details. Photograph of gingival fibroma is provided in Fig. 1.119.

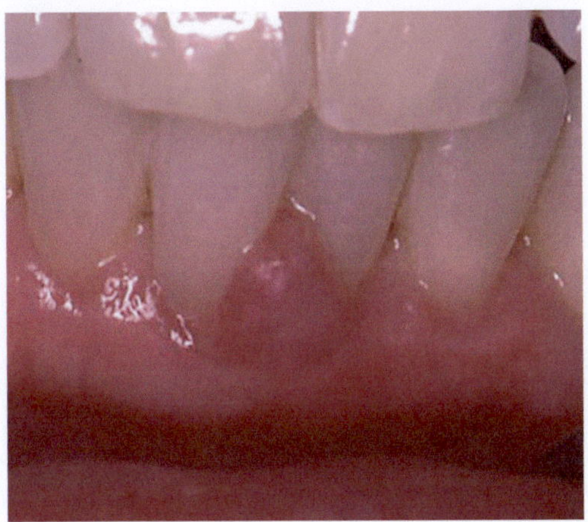

Fig. 1.119 Fibroma. Pink sessile nodule of the mandibular facial gingiva. The clinical differential diagnosis was fibroma versus peripheral ossifying fibroma (see pg 84)

Fibroma, Giant Cell Variant

There is a variant of fibroma referred to as a giant cell type fibroma. The clinical appearance is similar to a traditional fibroma except the surface can appear somewhat bosselated or papillary. It has a predilection for the gingiva and is not thought to be caused by chronic irritation or trauma. Treatment is surgical excision.

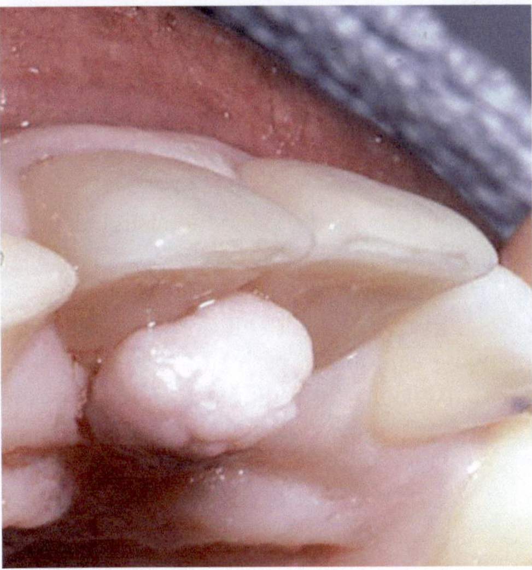

Fig. 1.120 Fibroma, giant cell type. Pink sessile nodule of the maxillary lingual gingiva

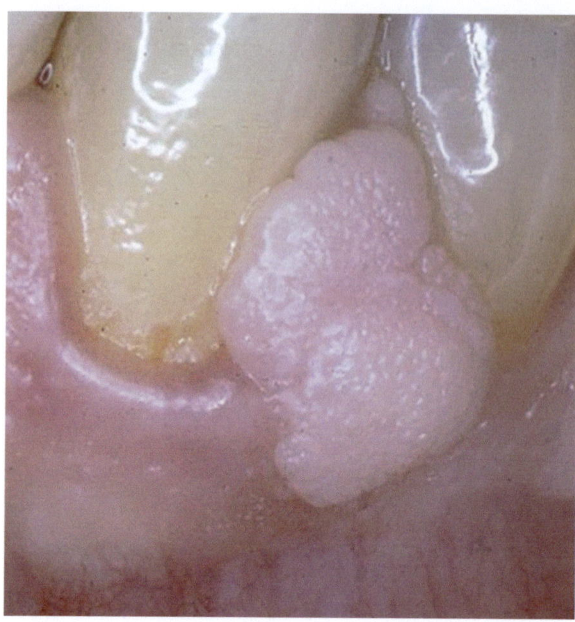

Fig. 1.121 Fibroma, giant cell type. Pink sessile nodule of the mandibular facial gingiva. Microscopic diagnosis was *fibroma, giant cell type*. Note the slight papillary appearance of the surface, which might cause the clinician to suspect papilloma or condyloma

Clinical Note The *retrocuspid papilla* is a circumscribed nodule located on the lingual anterior gingiva usually in the area of mandibular cuspids. This entity is observed more frequently in children and may regress with age. The retrocuspid papilla is considered to be a normal anatomical variation.

Peripheral Ossifying Fibroma

Clinical appearance: Non-painful, sessile or pedunculated, smooth, pink or red, nodule. Surface ulceration is not uncommon. Most commonly occurs in adolescents.

Etiology: Derived from cells of the periodontal ligament and thought to be a reactive lesion rather than a neoplasm.

Location: Occurs on the gingiva only.

Differential diagnosis:Fibroma, giant cell fibroma, if ulcerated and inflamed it could resemble pyogenic granuloma or peripheral giant cell granuloma.

Treatment: Surgical excision. In addition, any predisposing factors such as plaque or irritation should be removed. Recurrence is not uncommon and reportedly between 15 and 20%.

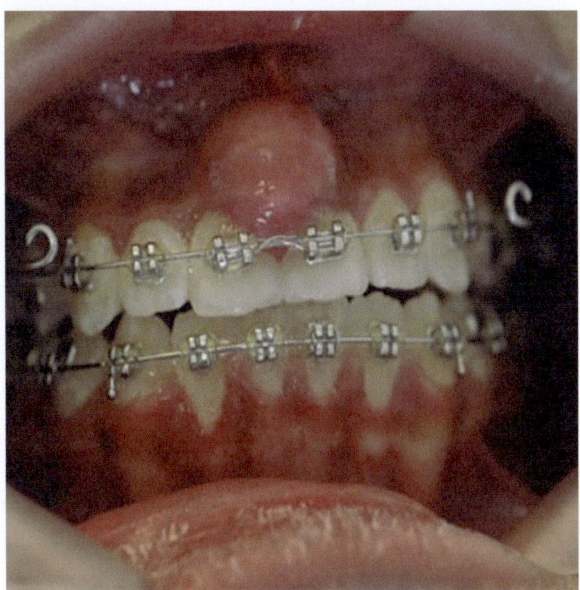

Fig. 1.122 Peripheral ossifying fibroma. Smooth surfaced, pink nodular mass of the maxillary anterior facial gingiva. *Photo courtesy of Dr. David Koslovsky, New York, NY*

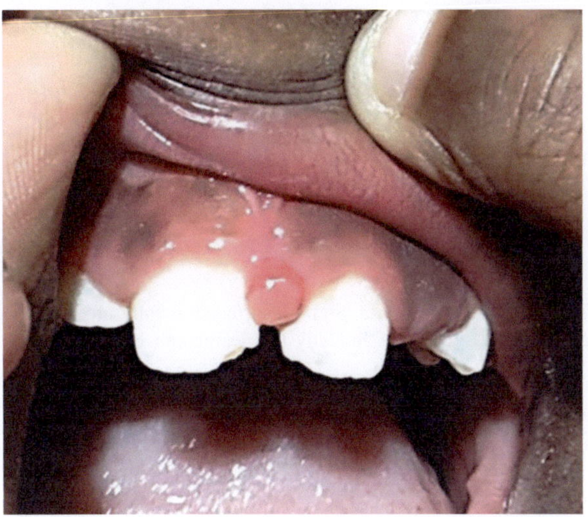

Fig. 1.123 Peripheral ossifying fibroma. Small smooth surfaced, centrally ulcerated pink-red nodule of the maxillary anterior facial gingiva

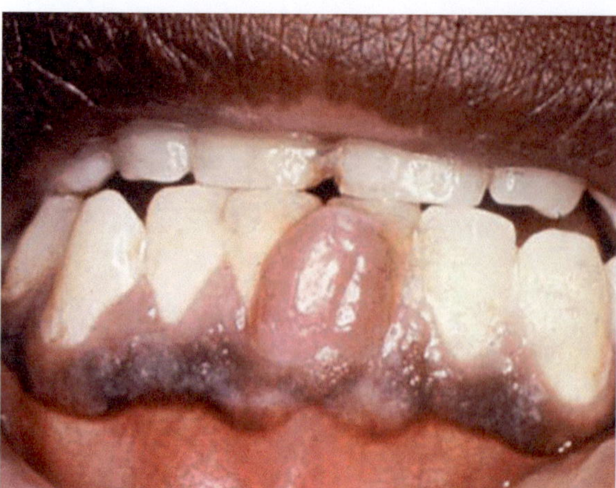

Fig. 1.124 Peripheral ossifying fibroma. Smooth surfaced, pink nodule of the mandibular anterior facial gingiva

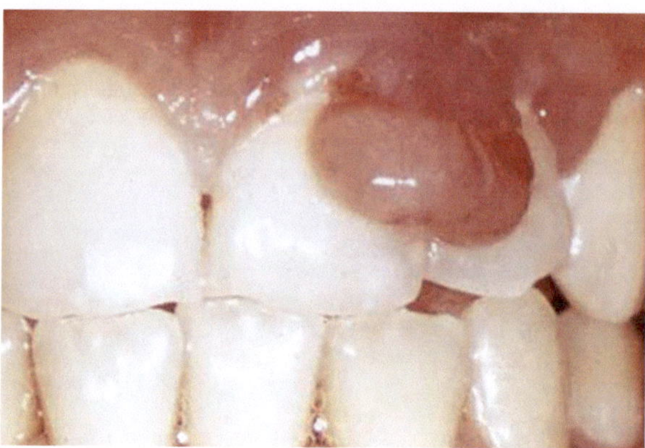

Fig. 1.125 Peripheral ossifying fibroma. Smooth surfaced, focally ulcerated pink-red nodule of the maxillary anterior facial gingiva. Clinically this lesion can be also interpreted as pyogenic granuloma

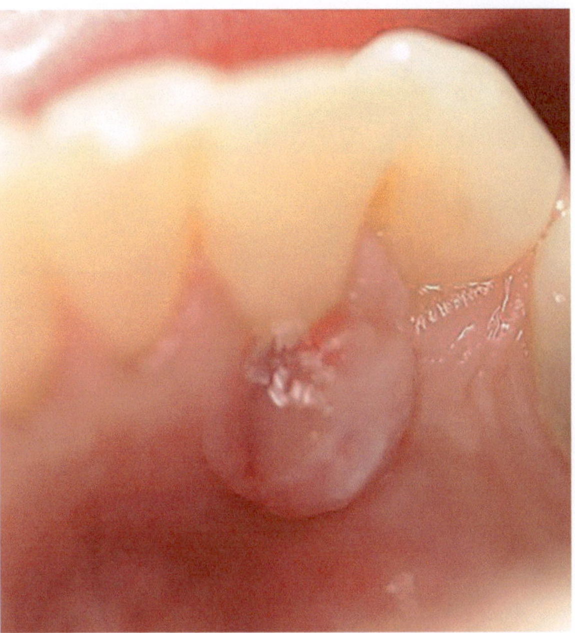

Fig. 1.126 Peripheral ossifying fibroma. Smooth surfaced, focally ulcerated pink-red nodule of the maxillary anterior lingual gingiva

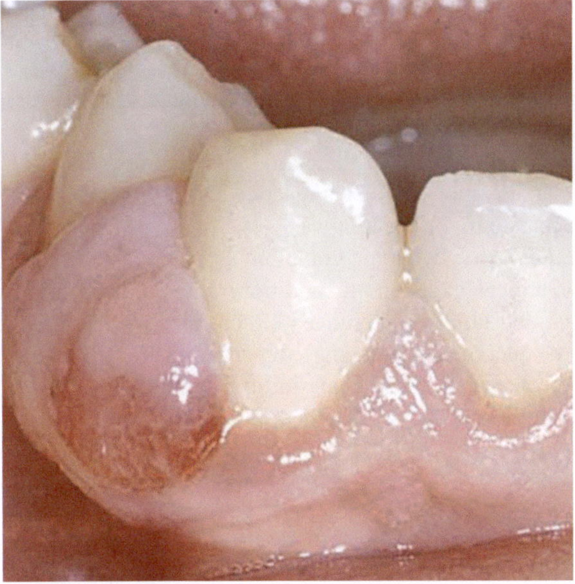

Fig. 1.127 Peripheral ossifying fibroma. Smooth surfaced, pink, and erythematous nodule of the mandibular anterior facial gingiva

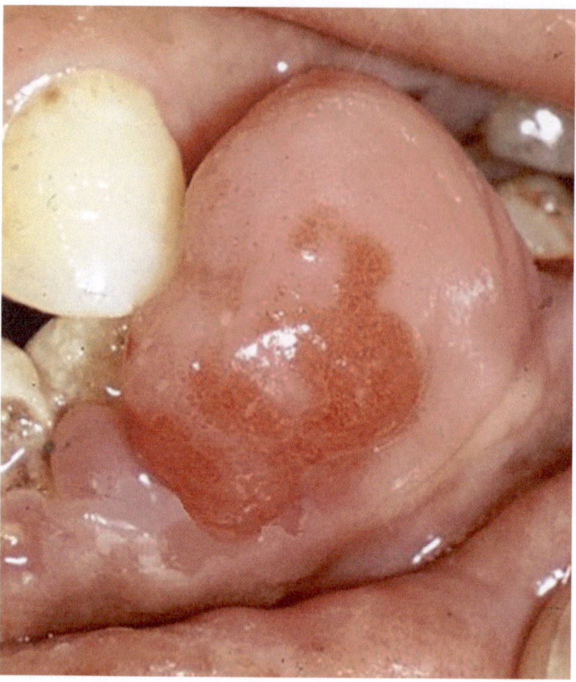

Fig. 1.128 Peripheral ossifying fibroma. Large smooth surfaced, pink-red nodule of the mandibular facial gingiva

Peripheral Giant Cell Granuloma

Clinical appearance: Dusky red, exophytic nodule. Sessile or pedunculated. Non-painful.

Etiology: Derived from cells of the periodontal ligament and, like the peripheral ossifying fibroma, it is thought to be a reactive lesion rather than a neoplasm.

Location: Occurs only on the gingiva.

Differential diagnosis: Pyogenic granuloma, peripheral ossifying fibroma.

Treatment: Surgical excision. In addition, any predisposing factors such as plaque or irritation should be removed. Recurrence is not likely but possible. Recurrence is not uncommon and reportedly around 18%. In pediatric patients with peripheral giant cell granuloma, the possibility of central involvement (central giant cell lesion/granuloma) should be excluded radiographically.

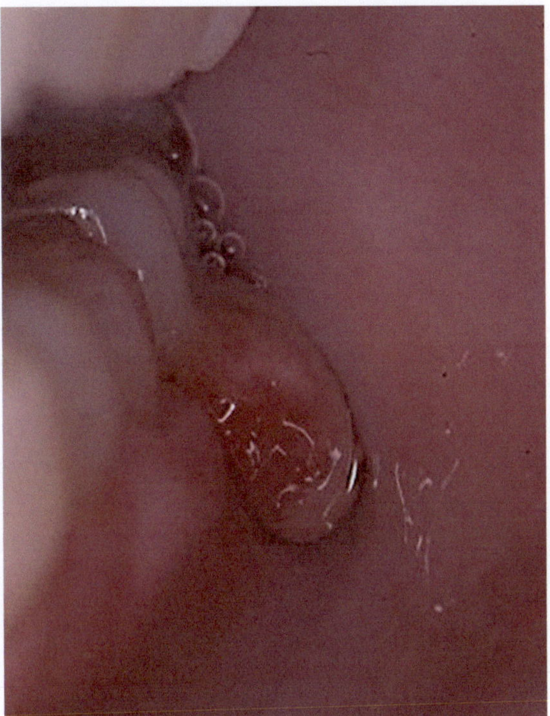

Fig. 1.129 Peripheral giant cell granuloma. Smooth surfaced, pink-red, nodule of the mandibular buccal gingiva. Patient is an adult

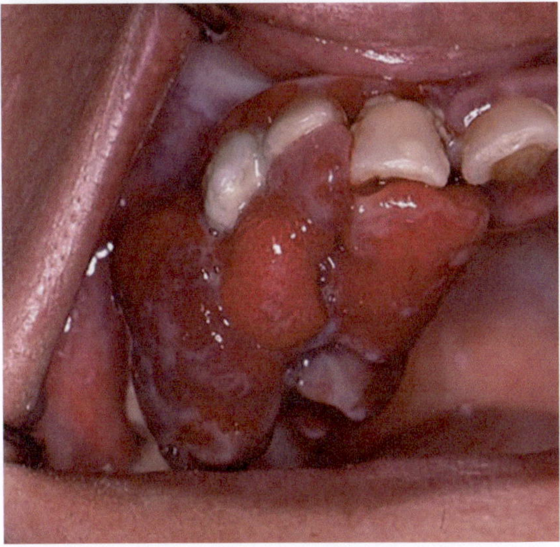

Fig. 1.130 Peripheral giant cell. Large, lobulated dusky red mass of maxillary gingiva. Patient is an adult

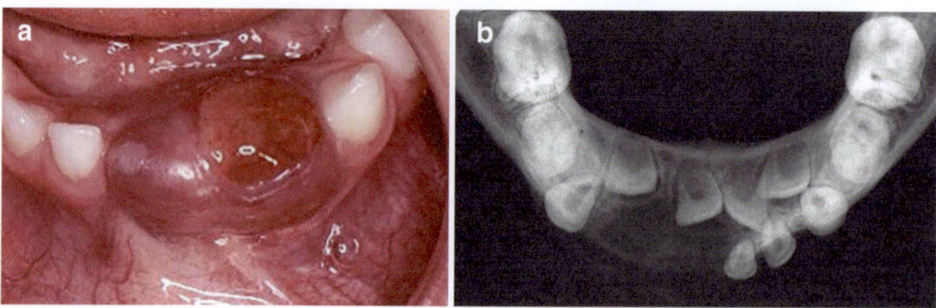

Fig. 1.131 (**a, b**) *Central giant cell granuloma* presenting a smooth surfaced, slightly dusky, ulcerated mass of the anterior mandibular gingiva of a 3-year-old child. An occlusal radiograph revealed an intra-osseous component of the tumor and the premature exfoliation if the right mandibular primary central and lateral incisors

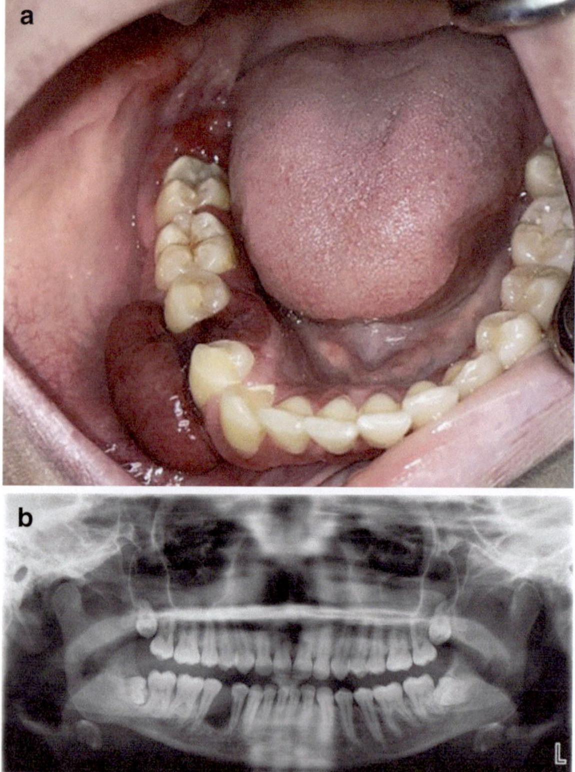

Fig. 1.132 (**a, b**) *Central giant cell granuloma* presenting a smooth surfaced, dusky red mass involving the buccal, interproximal and lingual gingiva. Radiographic examination of the lesion revealed an intra-osseous component

Note The above two cases illustrate the need for radiograph examination when a patient presents with a gingival mass

Eruption Cyst

Clinical appearance: A soft tissue swelling that occurs over an erupting tooth. Can appear bluish in color. Contains either clear fluid or blood. If filled with blood, it is also referred to as *eruption hematoma*.

Etiology: Soft tissue analogue of the dentigerous cyst, thought to arise from the separation of the epithelium from the enamel of the crown of the tooth due to an accumulation of fluid or blood in a dilated follicular space.

Location: Alveolar ridge overlying an erupting tooth.

Differential diagnosis: Clinical presentation is often diagnostic. A radiograph can confirm the presence of the associated erupting tooth.

Treatment: Can disappear on its own but if it is causing discomfort or bleeding, surgical unroofing is indicated to expose the unerupted tooth.

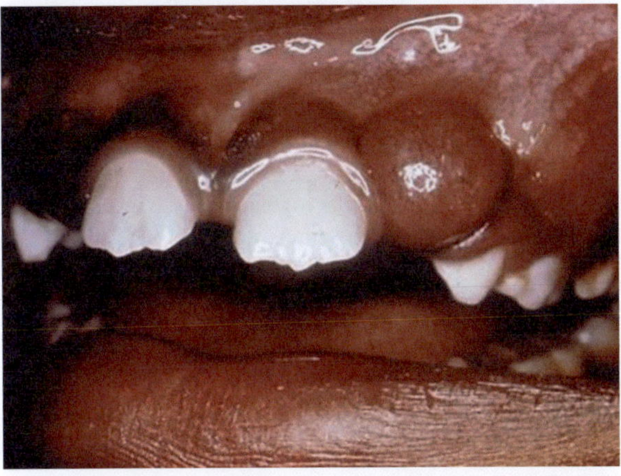

Fig. 1.133 Eruption cyst. Smooth surfaced, nodular swelling of the gingiva overlying an unerupted permanent maxillary lateral incisor

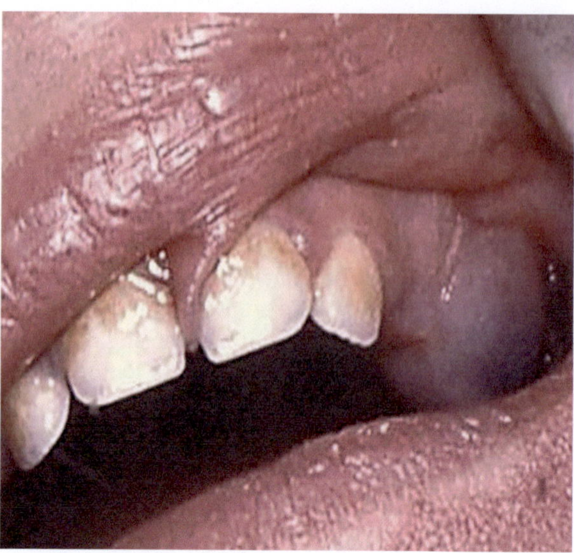

Fig. 1.134 Eruption hematoma. Smooth surfaced, blue-purplish nodular swelling of the gingiva overlying an unerupted primary maxillary molar

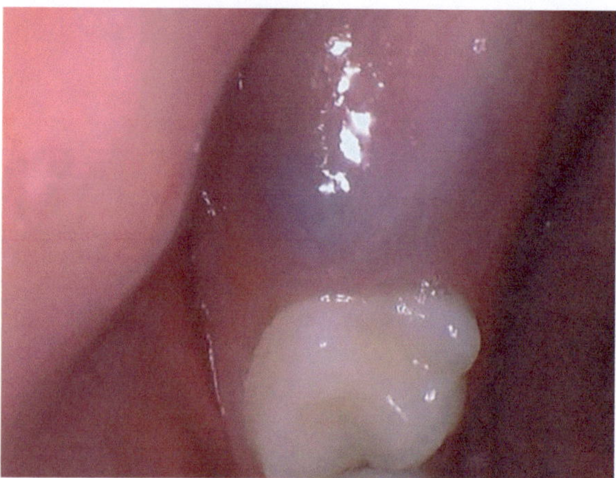

Fig. 1.135 Eruption cyst/hematoma. Smooth surfaced, blue-purplish nodular swelling of the gingiva overlying an unerupted first permanent maxillary molar. *Photo courtesy of Dr. Andrea Mann, Basking Ridge, NJ*

Parulis

Clinical appearance: Also called a gum boil, it is yellowish gingival swelling with associated erythema. The parulis is fluctuant when palpated and usually measures less than 5 mm in diameter. If a fistula is present pus can be expressed.

Etiology: A localized collection of pus in gingival soft tissue caused by necrosis of non-vital pulpal tissue or infected deep periodontal pocket (less likely in children).

Location: Gingiva adjacent to the apex of a non-vital tooth.

Differential diagnosis: Clinical and radiographic presentation is often diagnostic. Can appear clinically similar to a pyogenic granuloma, however, radiographic examination will reveal periapical pathosis. Histopathologically, abscess is present.

Treatment: Treating the source of infection (i.e., root canal therapy or extraction of offending tooth).

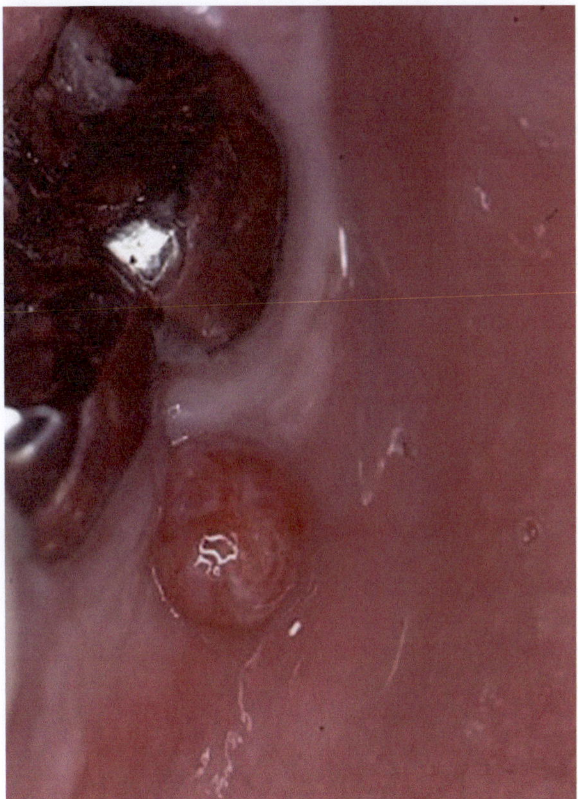

Fig. 1.136 Parulis. Yellow-red nodular swelling of the gingiva adjacent to apex of molar

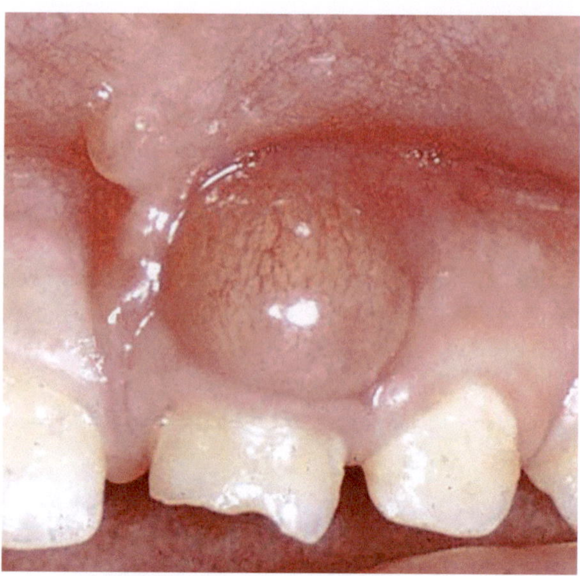

Fig. 1.137 Parulis. Yellow nodular swelling of the gingiva adjacent to fractured maxillary central incisor

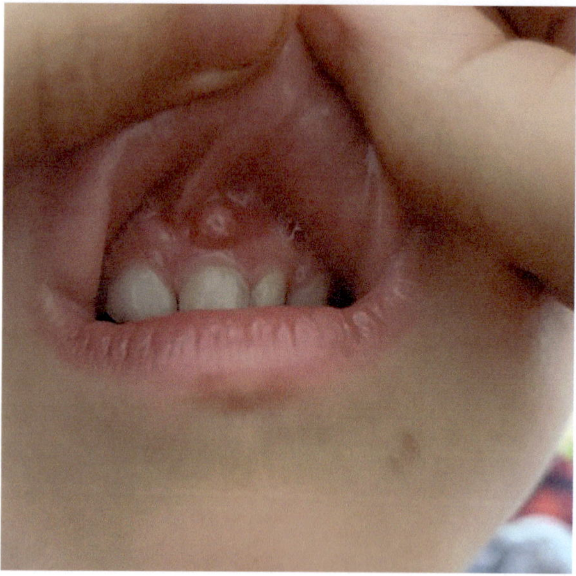

Fig. 1.138 Parulis. Yellow nodular swelling of the gingiva adjacent to apex of maxillary central incisor. Patient had history of trauma to the tooth. *Photo courtesy of Dr. Andrea Mann, Basking Ridge, NJ*

Summary of FOCAL GINGIVAL NODULES

Below is a summary of common diagnostic possibilities for a focal gingival nodule

Lesion	Clinical appearance	Other features
Pyogenic Granuloma	Red with a tendency to bleed	Most common in children and adolescents
Peripheral Ossifying Fibroma	Pink to red	Most common in adolescents
Fibroma/Giant Cell Fibroma	Pink	
Peripheral Giant Cell Granuloma	Dusky red	Can occur in children but most common in middle age/older adults
Eruption Cyst	Pink, overlying an unerupted tooth, can appear purple-blue as a result of secondary bleeding (eruption hematoma)	Periapical radiograph will reveal associated tooth
Parulis	Pink/yellowish, tends to be more apically located	Associated with a non-vital tooth and periapical radiolucency
Congenital Epulis[a]	Sessile or pedunculated pink to reddish mass of the anterior alveolar ridge in newborns	90% female predilection Can regress

[a]Congenital Epulis

Congenital epulis, also termed congenital granular cell tumor of infancy or the newborn, occurs on the anterior alveolar ridge. The maxilla is more often affected than the mandible and 90% of the infants with this lesion are females. The lesion presents as a smooth-surfaced sessile or pedunculated pink to reddish mass and can vary in size from several millimeters to a few centimeters. The lesion is benign and can undergo regression. Simple surgical excision is indicated if the lesion interferes with the baby's feeding or breathing.

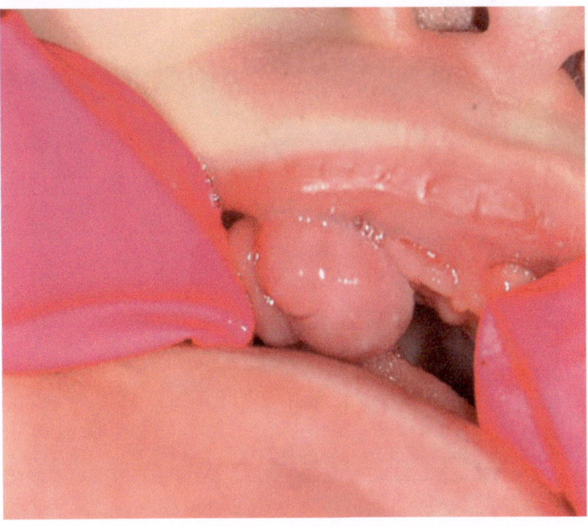

Fig. 1.139 Congenital epulis. Pink exophytic, slightly lobular growth of the edentulous maxillary alveolus in a female infant

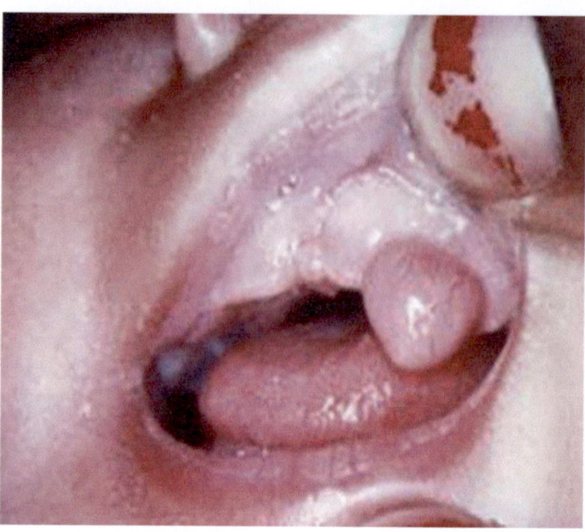

Fig. 1.140 Congenital epulis. Pink exophytic growth of the edentulous maxillary alveolus in a female infant

Gingival/Alveolar Cysts of the Newborn

Clinical appearance: Small (1–3 mm in diameter), white, keratin-filled bumps/papules located on the alveolar mucosa of newborns.

Etiology: Remnants of the dental lamina.

Location: Alveolar mucosa; maxilla more common than mandible.

Differential diagnosis: Bohn's nodules, Epstein's pearls; sometimes mistaken for natal teeth, but the position on the lateral ridge is inconsistent with the position of an erupting tooth.

Treatment: No treatment is necessary. Lesions spontaneously involute. Rarely seen in infants over 3 months of age.

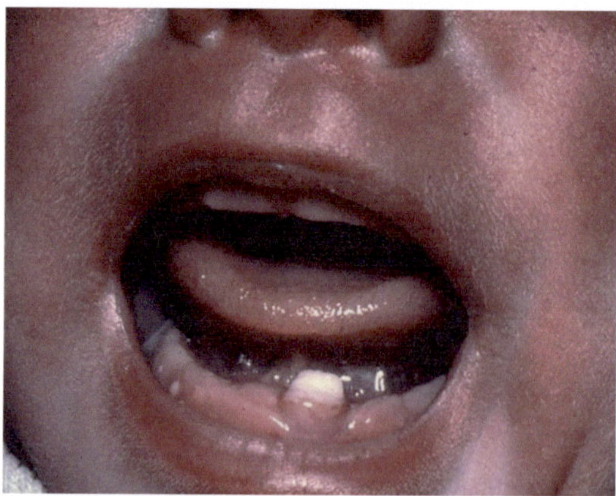

Fig. 1.141   Gingival cysts of newborn. Multiple small white papules on the right side of the edentulous mandibular alveolus in an infant

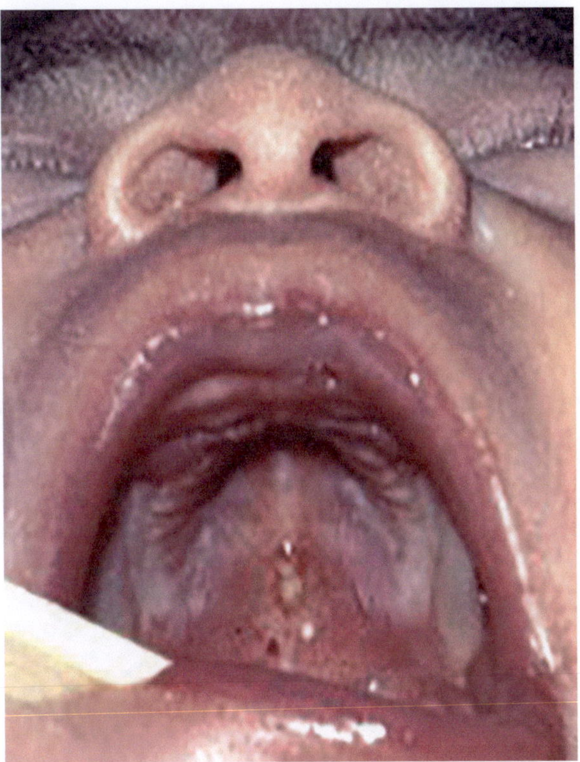

Fig. 1.142 Epstein's pearls. Multiple small white papules located along the median palatal raphe in an infant

Both *Epstein's pearls* and *Bohn's nodules* appear clinically identical to gingival cyst of newborns but differ in their locations. *Epstein's pearls* are located along the median palatal raphe and *Bohn's nodules* are scattered over the junction of the hard and soft palate. These terms are incorrectly used interchangeably in the literature

Localized Juvenile Spongiotic Gingival Hyperplasia

A recently recognized benign condition affecting the gingiva of children and young adults. Unlike conventional gingivitis, this entity does not respond to oral hygiene. Occasionally multifocal.

Clinical appearance: A localized area of erythema on the free and attached facial gingiva of anterior teeth, with a subtly papillary surface. The lesion is painless and often persistent.

Etiology: Unknown. One theory suggests that they arise from a localized area of ectopic junctional/sulcular epithelium in the free and attached gingiva.

Location: Facial gingiva of anterior teeth.

Differential diagnosis: Pyogenic granuloma, chronic hyperplastic gingivitis, peripheral giant cell granuloma.

- Chronic hyperplastic gingivitis is typically diffuse rather than focal; pyogenic granuloma is usually more exophytic; peripheral giant cell granuloma is duskier red in color, exophytic and not common in children.

Treatment: Since it is very uncommon in adults, localized juvenile spongiotic gingival hyperplasia is most likely a self-limited process and spontaneous remission does occur. Treatment has varied from no treatment to surgical excision. For persistent lesions, an incisional biopsy is appropriate to rule out other similar appearing lesions. Recurrence after excision has been reported in approximately 25% percent of cases.

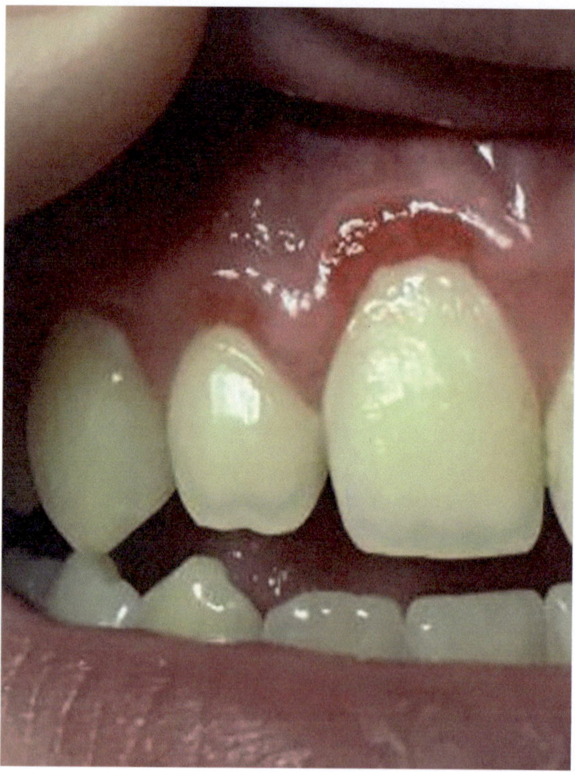

Fig. 1.143 Localized juvenile spongiotic gingival hyperplasia. Erythema localized to the free and attached facial gingiva of the maxillary central and lateral incisors

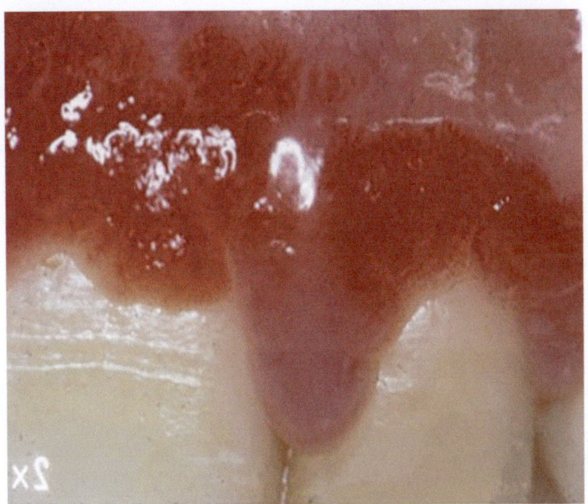

Fig. 1.144 Localized juvenile spongiotic gingival hyperplasia. Erythema with faint papillary appearance localized to the free and attached facial gingiva of the maxillary central and lateral incisors

Clinical Clue The focal nature—limited often to one or two teeth, can help discriminate localized spongiotic gingival hyperplasia from the more common plaque-induced or hormonal gingivitis which typically involves the gingiva of multiple teeth. Also, a close clinical examination reveals the red-involved gingiva to have a subtle papillary appearance.

Mouth-Breathing Gingivitis

Mouth breathing gingivitis is a unique form of hyperplastic gingivitis affecting the anterior facial gingiva in children and adolescents.

Clinical appearance: The gingiva appears swollen and red and can cover part of the crowns of the teeth. The most affected is the gingival tissue of maxillary anterior teeth. Bone loss and periodontal pocket formation can develop if oral hygiene is not well maintained.

Etiology: Mouth breathing. The gums become inflamed and hyperplastic because the mouth remains open. As a result, the mucosa is constantly exposed to the drying effect of air. The salivary flow has also decreased resulting in heavy plaque accumulation.

Location: Facial gingiva, the maxillary anterior is most commonly affected. In severe cases, it can be generalized.

Differential diagnosis: Medication/drug-induced gingival overgrowth, idiopathic gingival fibromatosis, hereditary gingival fibromatosis, leukemic infiltrate, granulomatosis with polyangiitis (formerly known as Wegener's granulomatosis; the use of this term is discouraged), and neurofibromatosis type I (von Recklinghausen's disease).

Evaluation of the medical history including the list of individual's medications is important in rendering the diagnosis. Mouth breathing can often be easily observed.

Treatment: Address the reason for mouth breathing (i.e., nasal obstruction and skeletal occlusion), oral hygiene improvement, elimination of causative factors and, in severe cases, gingivectomy. A biopsy is indicated in cases that do not respond to intervention. Lack of response to intervention could indicate a systemic disease, e.g., leukemic infiltrate (see below).

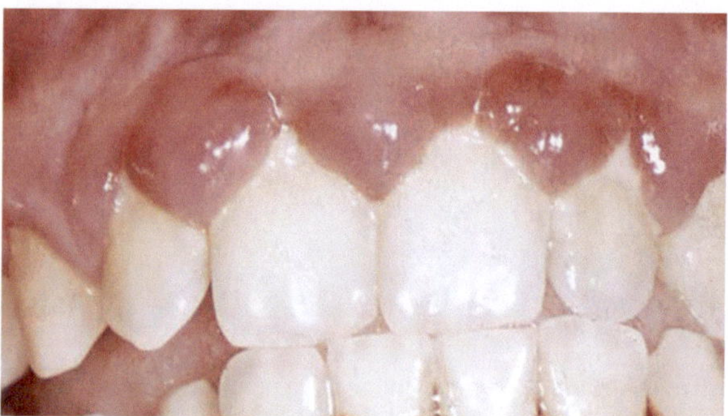

Fig. 1.145 Mouth breathing gingivitis. Swollen and erythematous maxillary gingiva. Note the plaque accumulation along the gingival margins and malocclusion

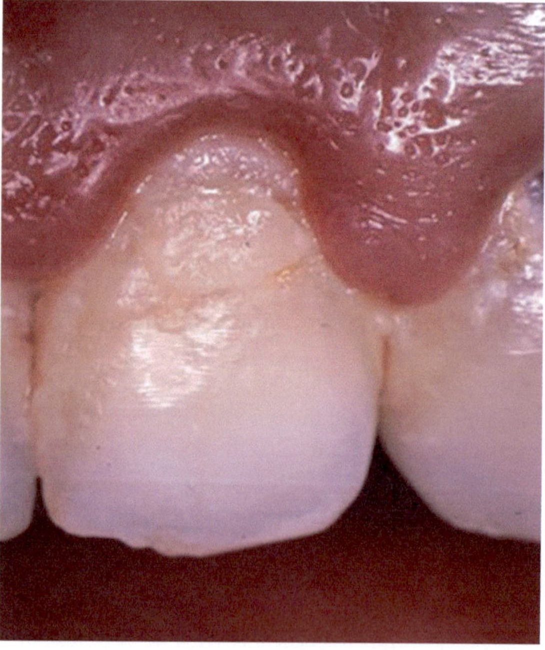

Fig. 1.146 Mouth breathing gingivitis. Swollen anterior maxillary gingiva with blunted papillae. Note the plaque accumulation

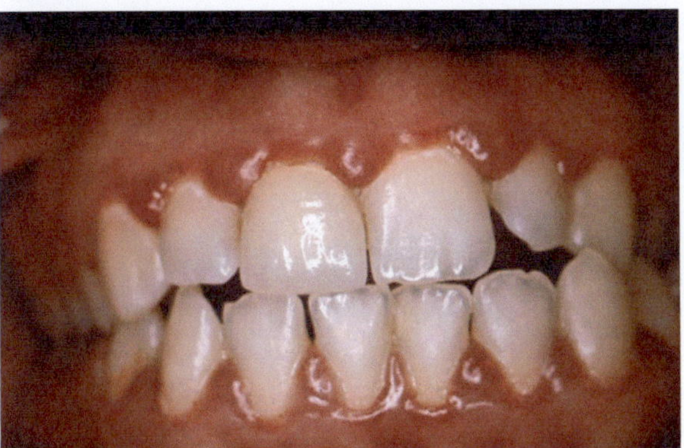

Fig. 1.147 Mouth breathing gingivitis. Swollen and erythematous anterior maxillary and mandibular gingiva with blunting of the papillae. Note the malocclusion

For comparison:

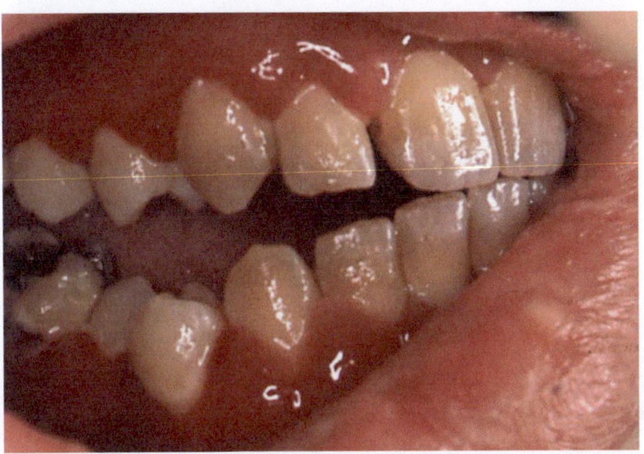

Fig. 1.148 Plaque-induced gingivitis. Erythema of the posterior marginal gingiva and less involvement of the anterior. Note the plaque accumulation on the mandibular premolrs and the decayed first molar

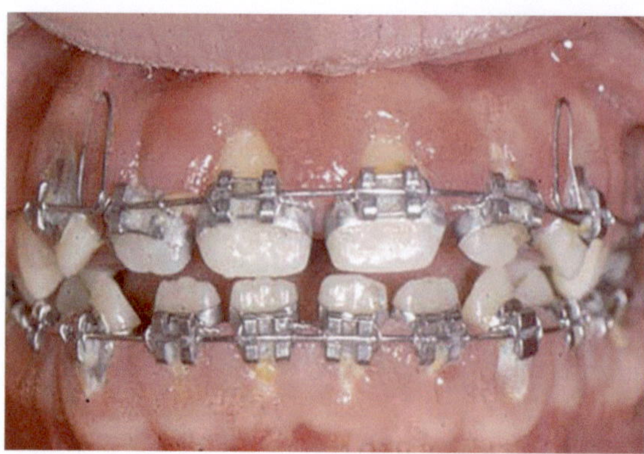

Fig. 1.149 *Hyperplastic gingivitis* resulting chronic irritation from the orthodontic bands and plaque accumulation

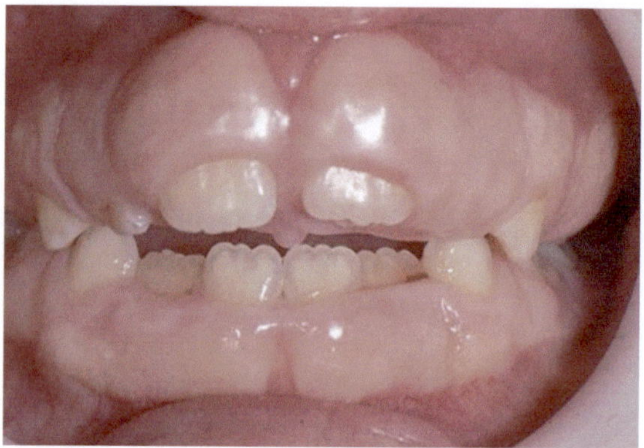

Fig. 1.150 Hereditary gingival fibromatosis. Pale pink generalized overgrowth of the gingiva

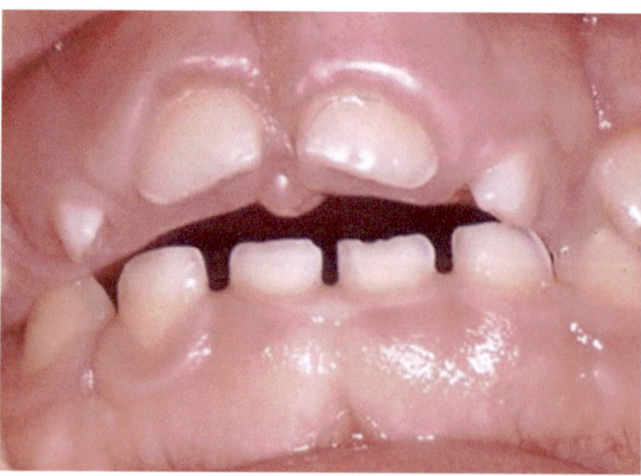

Fig. 1.151 Hereditary gingival fibromatosis. Pale pink generalized overgrowth of the gingiva

Hereditary gingival fibromatosis is the most common *syndromic* gingival enlargement in children. This autosomal dominant disease usually appears at the time of eruption of permanent dentition.

Medications such as phenytoin, nifedipine, and cyclosporine can cause gingival overgrowth. In addition, abuse of anabolic steroids has also been implicated in gingival overgrowth.

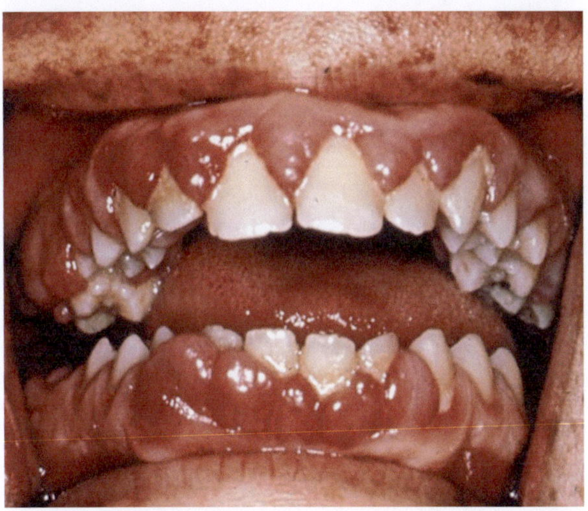

Fig. 1.152 Medication (Dilantin)-induced gingival overgrowth.** Generalized overgrowth of the gingiva. The erythema is secondary to poor oral hygiene

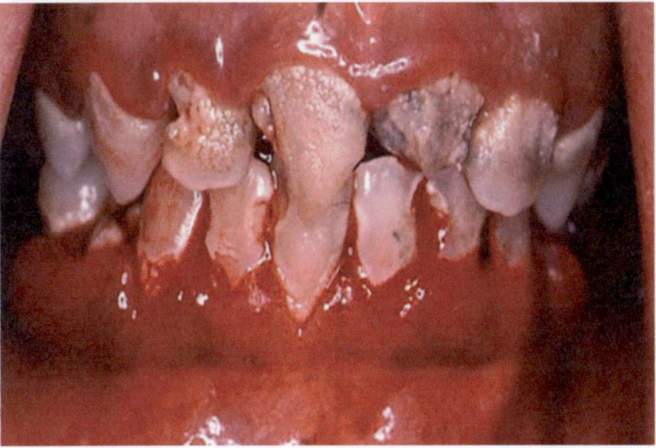

Fig. 1.153 Leukemic infiltrate. *** Swelling of the mandibular gingiva with spontaneous bleeding. Rampant decay and poor oral hygiene are also apparent

A leukemic infiltrate can also present as a gingival overgrowth (see Part II Oral Manifestations of Hematologic Diseases).

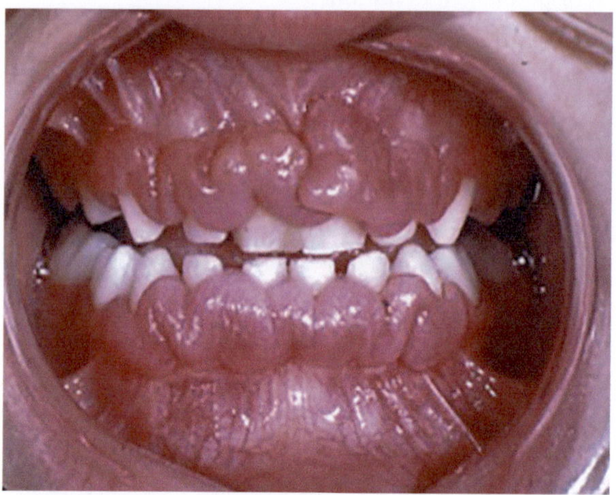

Fig. 1.154 Gingival hypertrophy in a child with *Juvenile hyaline fibromatosis (Murray–Puretic–Drescher syndrome)* is a rare, autosomal recessive disease that is characterized by abnormal growth of hyalinized fibrous tissue. The condition occurs from early childhood to adulthood. Clinical features include gingival hypertrophy/overgrowth, subcutaneous nodules, joint stiffness and contractures and muscle weakness

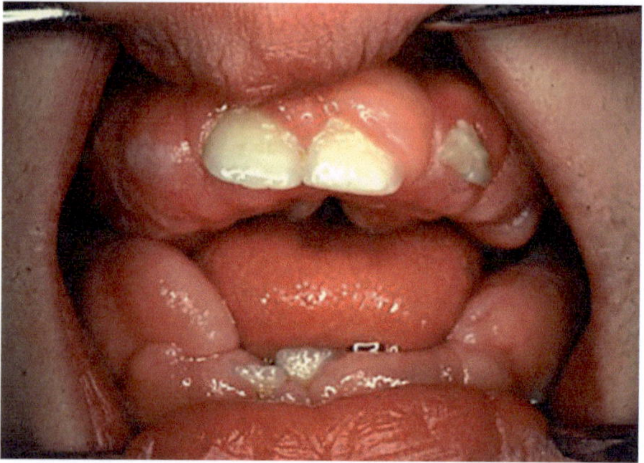

Fig. 1.155 Gingival overgrowth in a child with *Laband syndrome (Zimmerman-Laband syndrome)* is an rare autosomal recessive disorder characterized multiple congenital anomalies including gingival fibromatosis, coarse facial features, and absence or hypoplasia of nails or terminal phalanges of hands and feet

1.6 Pigmented Lesions

Pigmented lesions of the oral mucosa in children can be either exogenous or endogenous in origin. Examples of exogenous pigmentations include amalgam tattoo and pigmented hairy tongue. Endogenous pigmentations include focal or generalized melanosis and melanocytic nevi. Oral melanoma is *exceedingly rare* in children.

Medications can cause either exogenous or endogenous pigmentations. Exogenous pigmentation from medication results when the drug metabolite becomes deposited in the oral hard or soft tissue. An example of this is tetracycline staining. Endogenous pigmentation from medication results when the drug actually stimulates the production of melanin in oral mucosa. This type of medication-induced pigmentation might be seen in children with cancer who are receiving certain chemotherapeutic agents or in HIV-positive children being treated with AZT.

Depending on the type of the pigmented lesion, focal pigmentations include amalgam tattoos, melanotic macules, and melanocytic nevi. Diffuse pigmentations include physiologic pigmentation, pigmented hairy tongue, and medication-induced pigmentation.

The color also is variable depending on the source. In general, melanocytic lesions appear light to dark brown. Blue nevi appear gray-blue to bluish-black. Exogenous pigmentations vary depending on the agent responsible. The most common exogenous pigmentation, the amalgam tattoo, appears grayish blue to black. Graphite pigmentation, from the accidental traumatic embedding of pencil graphite in the oral mucosa demonstrates a similar appearance to an amalgam tattoo.

Pigmented Lesions
Amalgam tattoo
Melanotic Macule (Focal Melanosis)
Mucosal Nevi
Physiologic (Racial) Pigmentation

Amalgam Tattoo

Clinical appearance: Silver/gray, blue or black macule of the mucosa, often focal with either well-defined, irregular, or diffuse borders. Diagnosis is most often clinical based on appearance and history.

Etiology: Arise from iatrogenic implantation of amalgam particles or amalgam dust during the placement, polishing, or removal of amalgam fillings or during apicoectomies (uncommon in pediatric patients).

Location: Any mucosal tissue; floor of the mouth and gingiva/alveolar mucosa adjacent to an amalgam restoration are common locations.

Differential diagnosis: Melanotic macule, blue nevus, melanoma.

Treatment: Once diagnosis is established no treatment is necessary.

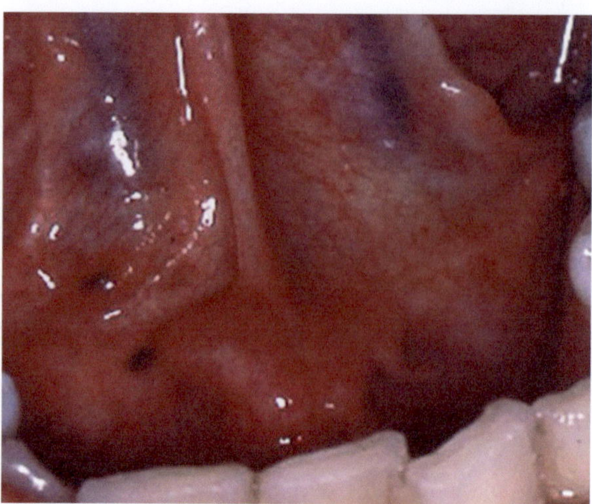

Fig. 1.156 Amalgam tattoo. Two lesions on the floor of mouth. Patient had amalgam restorations on the occlusal surfaces of the right and left mandibular first molars. Note the lingual veins for color comparison

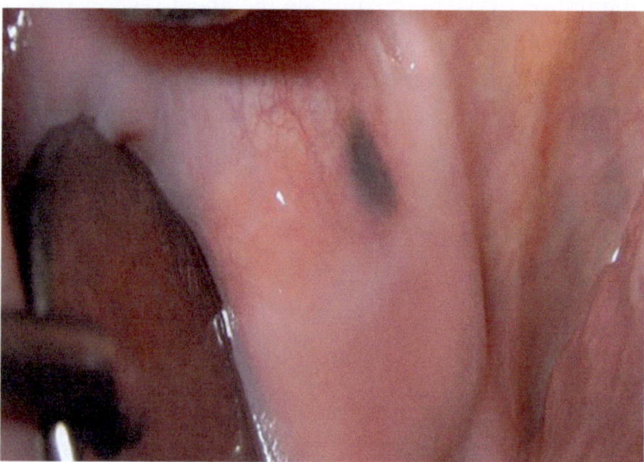

Fig. 1.157 Amalgam tattoo of the posterior buccal mucosa. Patient had amalgam restorations on the occlusal surface of the maxillary first molar

Clinical Note: The child must have a history of amalgam restoration, with the advent of composite restorations, the prevalence of amalgam tattoos will likely decrease.

Graphite pigmentation, from the accidental traumatic embedding of pencil graphite in the oral mucosa demonstrates a similar appearance to an amalgam tattoo.

Depending on the size of the embedded particles, some amalgam tattoos can be confirmed by radiograph.

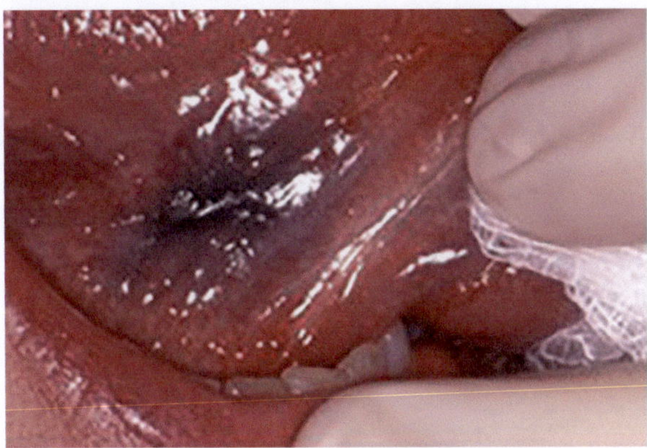

Fig. 1.158 Amalgam tattoo of the tongue. This amalgam tattoo is large with irregular and diffuse borders (in contrast to Fig 1.156). The patient had history of amalgam restorations on the occlusal and interproximal surfaces of the adjacent mandibular molar

Melanotic Macule (Focal Melanosis)

Clinical appearance: Brown to black macule of the mucosa, with well-defined borders, usually less than 7 mm; lesions are solitary but there can be more than one. More common in adults than in children.

Etiology: Oral equivalent of a cutaneous freckle, caused by an increase in melanin production. However, unlike a freckle, it is not related to sun exposure.

Location: Any mucosal tissue, usually gingiva, palate; those occurring on the lip vermillion are referred to as *labial melanotic macules.*

Differential diagnosis: Amalgam tattoo, nevus, melanoacanthoma, and melanoma.

Treatment: Once the diagnosis is established no treatment is needed.

Clinical Note
The size should be less than 7 mm, the color homogenous, the lesion flat and the size and color stable/unchanged.

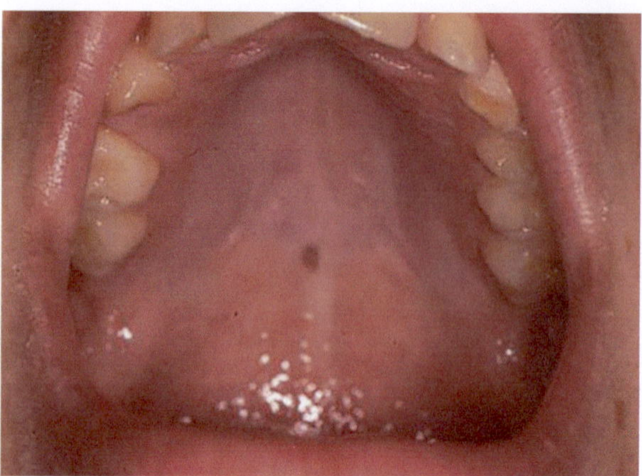

Fig. 1.159 Melanotic macule. Brown homogenous flat pigmentation of the palate in an 11-year-old male

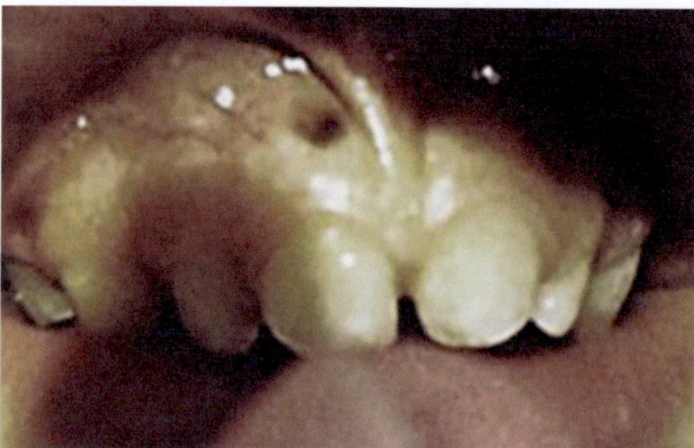

Fig. 1.160 Melanotic macule. Dark brown, flat pigmentation of the unattached gingiva in a 3-year-old child

Multifocal Perioral and Intraoral Melanotic Macules

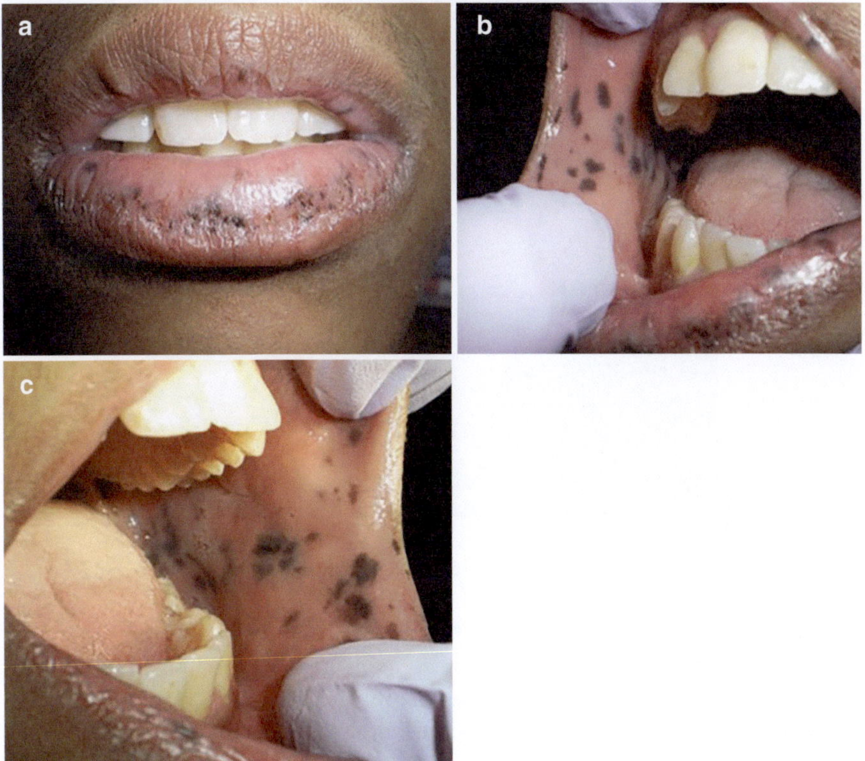

Fig. 1.161 (a–c) Multiple labial pigmentations and multifocal intraoral melanotic macules in a 12-year-old male. The lesions were present since infancy but were becoming more numerous according to parent. Patient was referred to geneticist and pediatric gastroenterologist for suspected *Peutz-Jeghers syndrome*

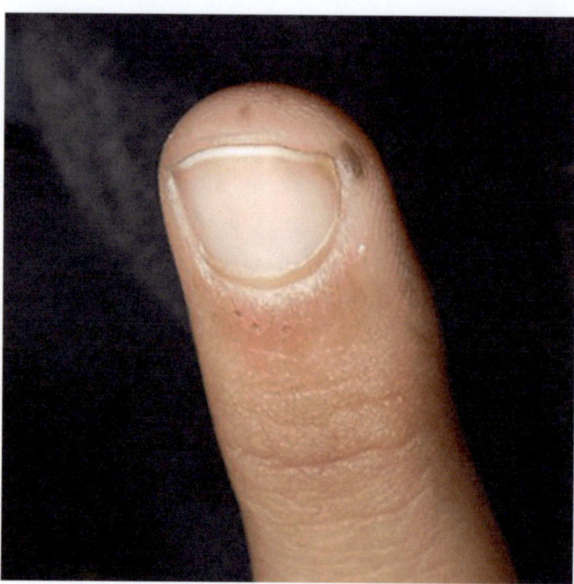

Fig. 1.162 Index finger of patient in Fig. 1.161. Note the presence of melanotic macules

Peutz-Jeghers syndrome is an autosomal dominant disease in which sufferers develop multiple benign hamartomatous polyps in the gastrointestinal tract and melanotic macules on the lips, oral mucosa, and skin of the hands and feet. *The oral pigmentations appear during the first year of life*, and therefore play an important role in early diagnosis. Although the GI polyps are generally benign, patients still have increased risk for the development of adenocarcinoma of the colon and rectum, as well as, increased risk for other malignancies including breast, pancreas, cervix, ovaries, and lung. Peutz–Jeghers syndrome has an incidence of approximately 1 in 25,000–300,000 births. The differential diagnosis of Peutz-Jeghers when it comes to perioral and oral melanotic macules includes Carney complex, also referred to as NAME (nevi, atrial myxoma, skin myxoma, ephelides) or LAMB (lentigines, atrial myxoma, mucocutaneous myxoma, blue nevus) syndrome.

Physiologic (Racial) Pigmentation

Clinical appearance: Multifocal or diffuse, light to dark brown pigmentated lesions of the oral mucosa which occurs in children with a darker complexion. Develops during the first two decades of life.

Etiology: Increased melanin production.

Location: Any mucosal tissue, especially on the attached gingiva.

Differential diagnosis: Nevus, melanoacanthoma, melanoma.

Treatment: Once diagnosis is established no treatment is needed.

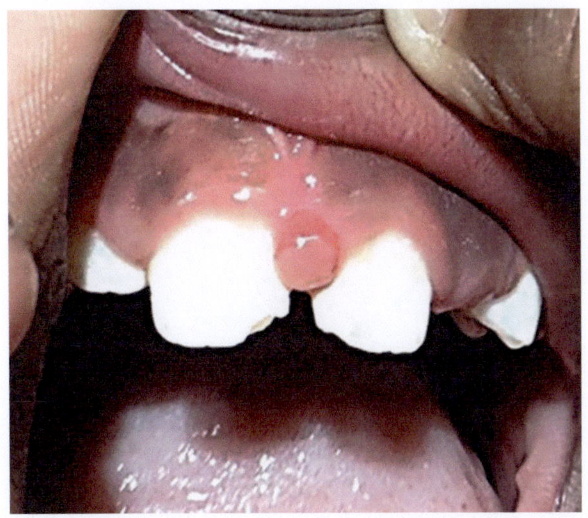

Fig. 1.163 Physiologic pigmentation. Diffuse brown pigmentation of the gingiva in a 7-year old with an ulcerated gingival nodule (peripheral ossifying fibroma)

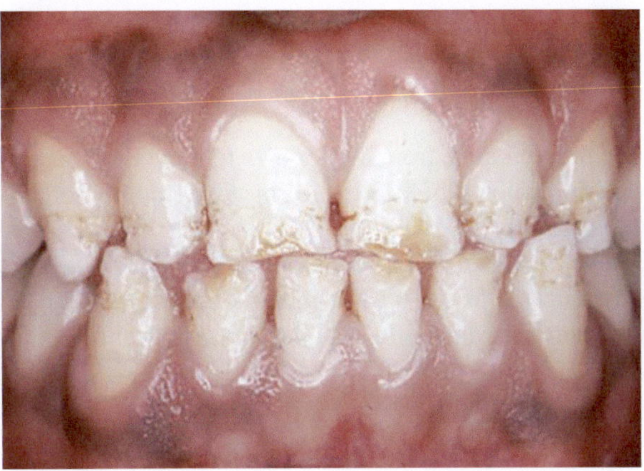

Fig. 1.164 Physiologic pigmentation. Diffuse light brown physiologic pigmentation of the gingiva in a 16-year old with mottled enamel

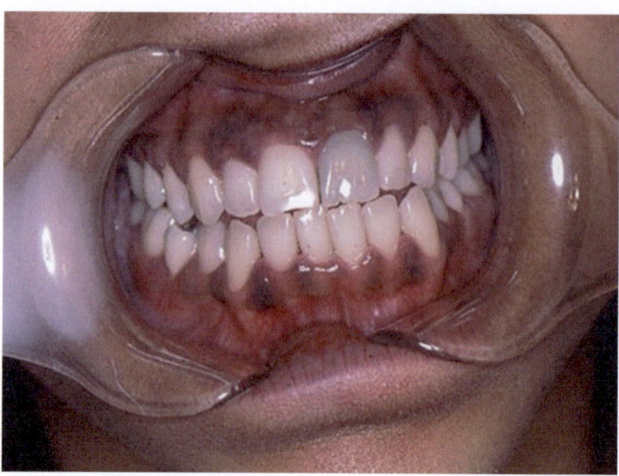

Fig. 1.165 Physiologic pigmentation. Diffuse dark brown physiologic pigmentation of the gingiva in an adolescent. Note gray discoloration of non-vital central incisor. Patient had history of trauma to that tooth

Mucosal Nevi

Unlike cutaneous nevi, oral nevi are rare but are commonly included in the differential diagnosis of oral pigmented lesions. Mucosal nevi can be either congenital or acquired and are microscopically classified as junctional, intramucosal, compound, and blue.

Clinical appearance: Range from light brown to blue/black and can be either flat or dome-shaped. The color should be uniform with smooth borders and stable in size with an intact surface.

Etiology: Benign proliferation of nevus cells.

Location: Any mucosal tissue, most common on the gingiva and hard palate.

Differential diagnosis: Melanotic macule, amalgam tattoo, melanoacanthoma, melanoma.

Treatment: Once the diagnosis is established with biopsy, no further treatment is needed.

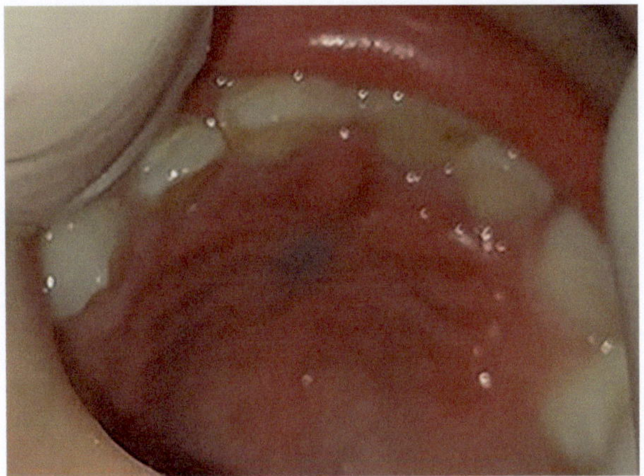

Fig. 1.166   Blue nevus. Focal blue-gray pigmentation of the hard palate in a 3-year old

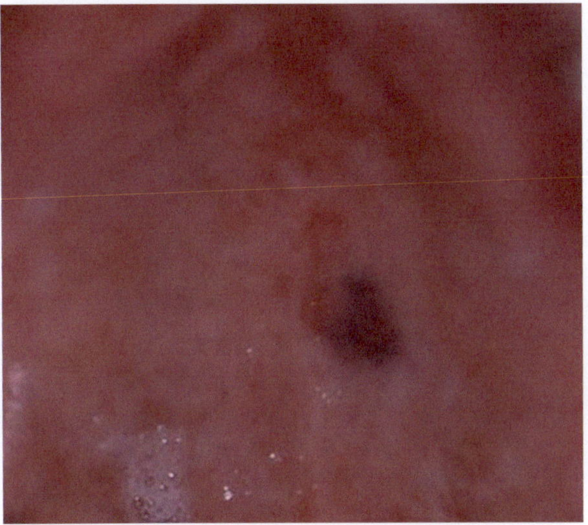

Fig. 1.167   Blue nevus. Focal blue-gray pigmentation of hard palate

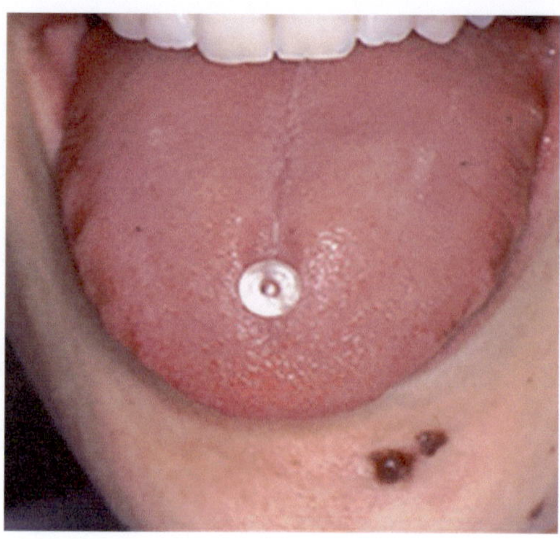

Fig. 1.168 Cutaneous nevi. Brown pigmented cutaneous nevi of the chin in teenager with a tongue piercing

Coated Tongue

Clinical appearance: Diffuse white to brown-black appearance of the dorsal tongue.

Etiology: Hypertrophy or lack of desquamation of the filiform papillae with secondary exogenous staining from food, beverages (chlorhexidine digluconate).

Location: Tongue dorsum.

Differential diagnosis: Usually clinically diagnostic.

Treatment: Gentle tongue brushing, staying hydrated, and avoiding alcohol-containing mouthwash

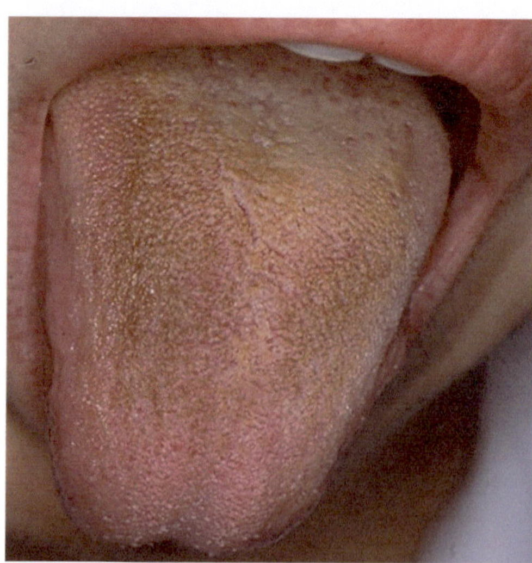

Fig. 1.169 Brown coated/hairy tongue. Diffuse light brown discoloration of the dorsal tongue

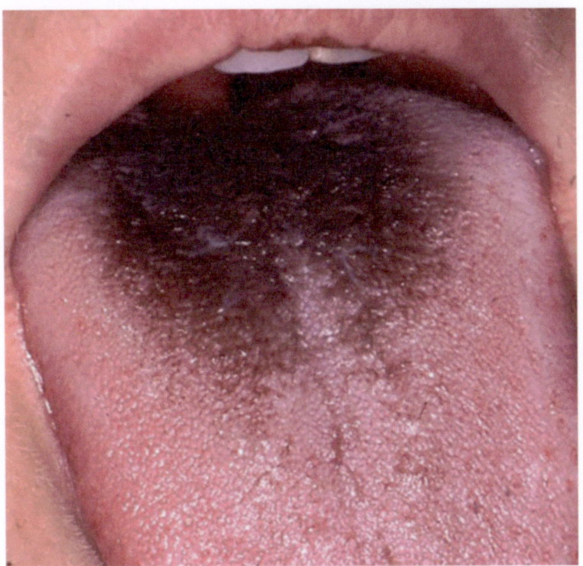

Fig. 1.170 Brown coated/hairy tongue. Dark brown discoloration of the posterior dorsal tongue

Mucosal Manifestations of Systemic Disease, Habits and Abuses

2

2.1 Mucosal Manifestations of Gastrointestinal Disease

Gastrointestinal (GI) disorders—including celiac disease, irritable bowel syndrome (IBS), and inflammatory bowel disease (i.e., ulcerative colitis and Crohn's disease) can present with intraoral manifestations. Oral manifestations of GI disease are more common in children compared to adults. In some cases, particularly with Crohn's disease, the oral lesions can present in the setting of subclinical GI symptoms or can even present several months to years before any GI manifestations. Oral lesions preceding gastrointestinal manifestations of Crohn's disease can be seen in as much as 60% of patients.

1. Recurrent aphthous stomatitis-like ulcerations

   Recurrent aphthous stomatitis-like ulcers can be seen in patients with malabsorption syndromes such as celiac disease as well as patients with IBS, ulcerative colitis, and Crohn's disease.

> Any patient presenting with a history of recurrent aphthae or aphthous-like ulcers should be questioned about GI symptoms—namely: GI discomfort, bloating, constipation, and diarrhea.

2. Pyostomatitis Vegetans

   Pyostomatitis vegetans is characterized by erythematous, thickened oral mucosa with multiple pustules, and superficial erosions. It is a manifestation of inflammatory bowel disease, most commonly seen in patients with ulcerative colitis.

© The Author(s), under exclusive license to Springer Nature Switzerland AG 2023
E. Philipone et al., *Oral Pathology in the Pediatric Patient*,
https://doi.org/10.1007/978-3-031-30900-7_2

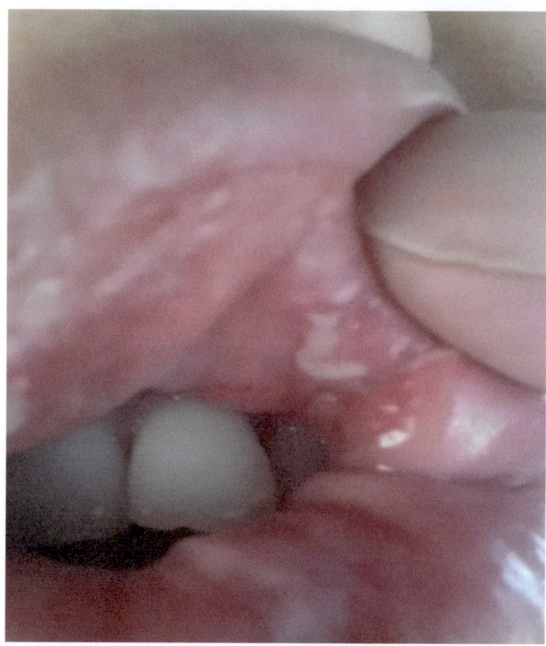

Fig. 2.1 *Pyostomatitis vegetans* "snail track" mucosal pustules with associated erythema of the upper lip mucosa

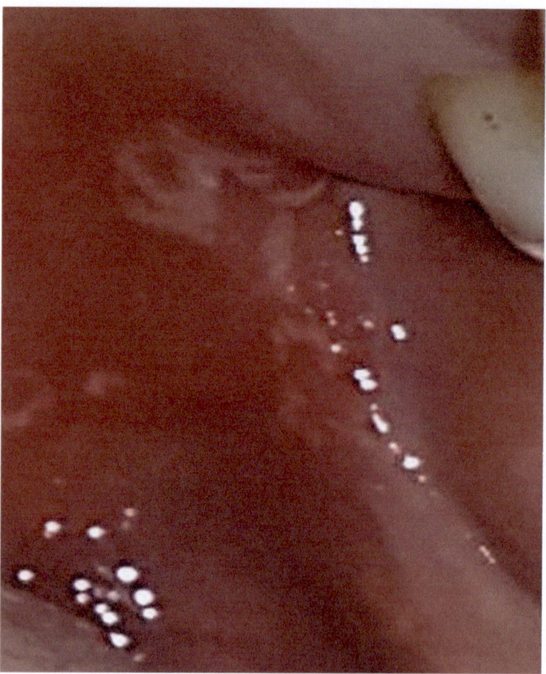

Fig. 2.2 *Pyostomatitis vegetans* "snail track" mucosal pustules with erythema of the soft palate

3. Mucosal Tags or Folds

   Mucosal tags or folds in the labial and buccal vestibules and in the retromolar mucosa are associated with Crohn's disease. Up to 75% of these lesions may show non-caseating granulomas on histopathology.

4. Cobblestoning

   In patients with Crohn's disease, the posterior buccal mucosa and mucobuccal folds can become swollen and fissured with a corrugated and hyperplastic appearance.

5. Mucogingivitis

   The gingiva may become edematous, granular, and hyperplastic in patients with Crohn's disease. The entire attached gingiva down to the mucogingival junction can be affected.

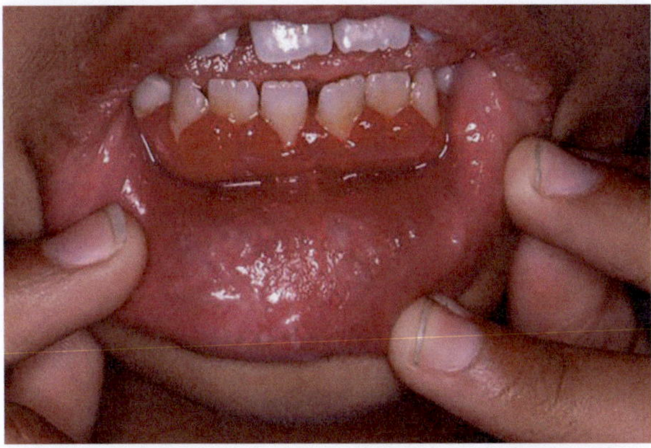

Fig. 2.3 Mucogingivitis. Edematous and erythematous, hyperplastic gingiva in a 8-year old with Crohn's disease. Focally, the involvement extends to the mucogingival junction

6. Persistent Orofacial Swelling (Orofacial Granulomatosis)

   Orofacial granulomatosis is an uncommon inflammatory disorder that involves the orofacial region, most commonly presenting as a persistent swelling in one or both lips. Orofacial granulomatosis has been documented to be one of the initial presentations of Crohn's disease. Children who develop orofacial granulomatosis under the age of 16 years are more likely to develop Crohn's disease compared to those over the age of 16 years. Therefore, the initial presentation of orofacial granulomatosis in the pediatric population, in the absence of other causes, warrants careful long-term evaluation for Crohn's disease. In these patients, management of the GI condition usually results in the resolution of the oral manifestations.

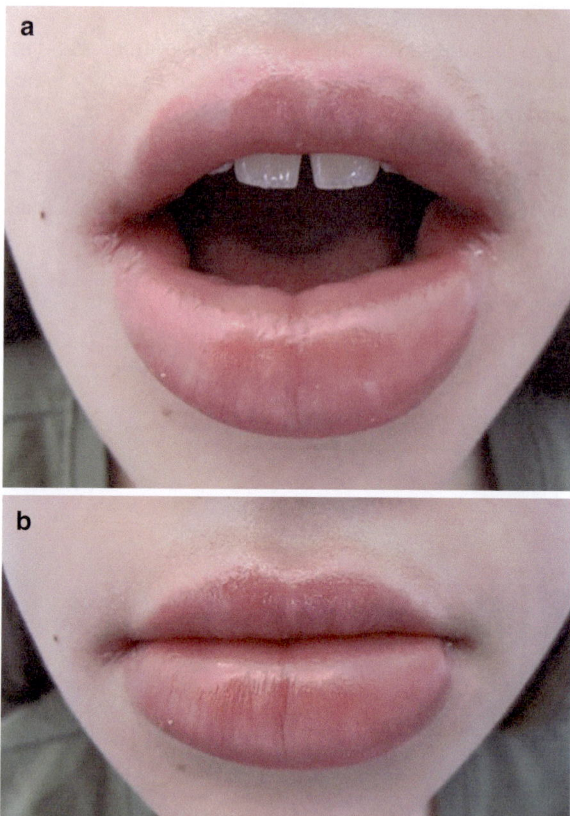

Fig. 2.4 (**a**, **b**) Orofacial granulomatosis. 12-year old with persistent, non-tender lower lip swelling. The patient denied any GI symptoms. A biopsy revealed granulomatous inflammation. Patient subsequently developed GI symptoms 2 years later and was diagnosed with Crohn's disease

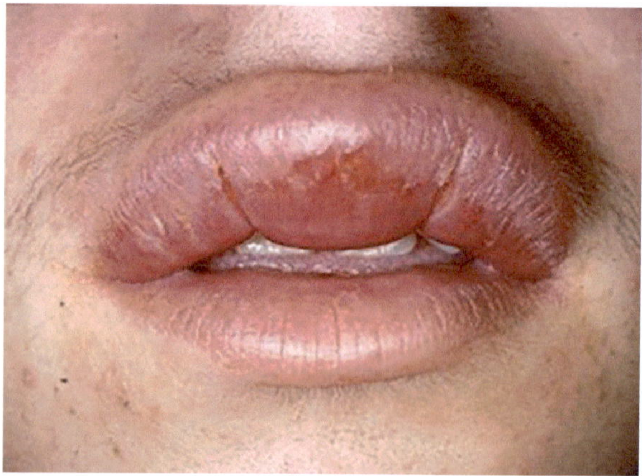

Fig. 2.5 Orofacial granulomatosis. Persistent, non-tender upper lip swelling

Conditions that can mimic Orofacial granulomatosis:
- Hypersensitivity reaction to cinnamon, benzoate, dental products
- Chronic granulomatous disease
- Sarcoidosis
- Tuberculosis
- Granulomatosis with polyangiitis

Screening tests to rule out these other entities should be considered.

Clinical Note Orofacial granulomatosis can clinically mimic *angioedema*. However, a distinguishing feature is the duration of the swelling. Orofacial granulomatosis is a persistent swelling whereas in angioedema the swelling lasts minutes to hours and can be itchy or painful with urticaria occurring concurrently. It is also important to note that angioedema could be a medical emergency if the swelling involves the throat. In children, angioedema can be the result of an allergy, idiopathic, or inherited.

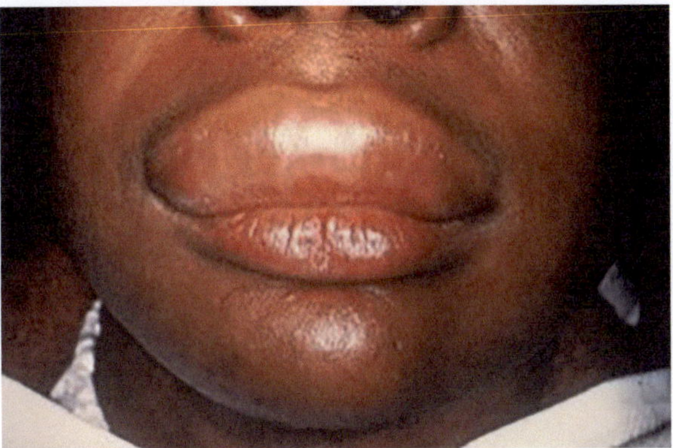

Fig. 2.6 Angioedema. Transient, non-tender upper lip swelling

2.2   Mucosal Manifestations of Nutritional Deficiencies

The cause of nutritional deficiencies is either from decreased intake (i.e., a diet that lacks essential nutrients) or the inability to absorb the nutrients (i.e., gastrointestinal conditions such as celiac disease). Children are more at risk for serious complications due to nutritional deficiencies than adults. Nutritional deficiencies affect children of all socio-economic backgrounds but are more frequently seen in children from financially disadvantaged families and in children with underlying systemic diseases. In many cases nutritional deficiencies show intraoral manifestations. Although deficiencies can affect teeth, periodontal tissues, as well as salivary glands, for the purpose of this atlas, we will focus on the mucosal manifestations.

Iron Iron deficiency can result in anemia. As in the various forms of anemias, the oral manifestations of iron-deficiency anemia include mucosal pallor, most notable on the gingiva and lips, angular cheilitis, and atrophic glossitis (loss of papillae of the dorsal tongue, resulting in a smooth red appearance). Patients may complain of glossodynia or dysphagia. Iron deficiency is also a predisposing factor for oral candidiasis. Patients also might suffer from recurrent bouts of aphthous stomatitis.

According to the WHO, approximately 40% of preschool children in developing countries are estimated to suffer from iron-deficiency anemia. In many developing countries, iron deficiency is caused by parasite infections, e.g., malaria and other infectious diseases such as HIV and tuberculosis.

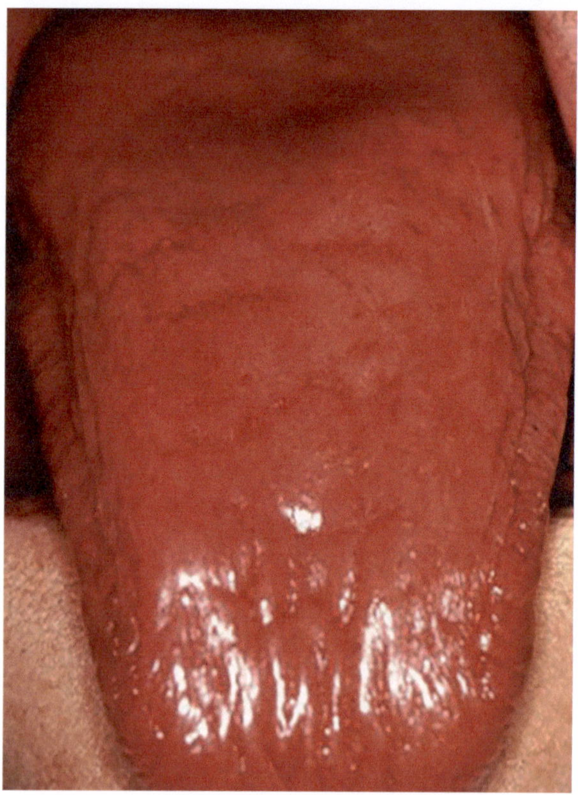

Fig. 2.7 Atrophic glossitis. Smooth/bald dorsal tongue with erythema

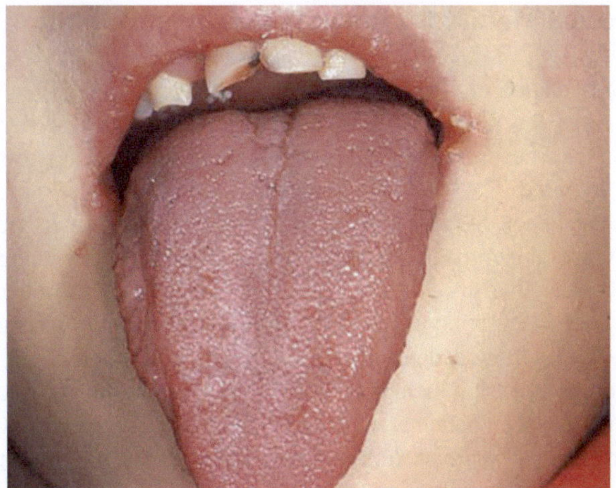

Fig. 2.8 Angular cheilitis. Cracking at the corners of the mouth

Vitamin A   Vitamin A deficiency can result in impaired healing, desquamation of the oral mucosa, keratosis, decreased taste sensitivity, xerostomia, and increased risk for candidiasis.

Riboflavin (Vitamin B$_2$), Niacin (Vitamin B$_3$), Pyridoxine (Vitamin B$_6$), and Folic Acid (Vitamin B9)   Vitamin B2, B3, B6, and B9 deficiencies can result in angular cheilitis, atrophic glossitis, increased risk of candidiasis, and glossodynia.

Cobalamin (Vitamin B$_{12}$)   Vitamin B$_{12}$ deficiency can result in *pernicious anemia*. Similar to the other B vitamins, oral manifestations include angular cheilitis, atrophic glossitis, increased risk of candidiasis, and glossodynia. Patients can also develop mucositis and complain of burning mouth. The tongue often is described as having a "beefy red" appearance. Patients can demonstrate aphthous-like ulcers, delayed wound healing, and xerostomia.

Vitamin C   Chronic vitamin C deficiency can result in scurvy. Patients present with red, swollen gingiva, periodontal disease, burning mouth, soft tissue ulcerations, and are at increased risk for candidiasis.

Vitamin K   Oral manifestations include increased bleeding, especially of the gingiva.

Clinical Note
Many of the signs and symptoms of vitamin deficiencies overlap and are non-specific, therefore a thorough evaluation of the patient's nutritional status is needed before initiating any isolated replacement therapy.

2.3   Mucosal Manifestations of Immunosuppression

The clinical presentation of oral lesions in immunosuppressed children is highly variable. In some cases, it is the oral manifestations that result in the discovery of an underlying condition that is causing the immunosuppression. Immunosuppression can either be primary or acquired. The World Health Organization recognizes more than 100 primary immune deficiency diseases. Examples include DiGeorge syndrome, complement deficiencies, X-linked gammaglobulinemia (Bruton's) disease, immunoglobulin heavy chain deficiency, selective IgA deficiency, transient hypogammaglobulinemia of infancy, phagocytic disorders, severe congenital neutropenia (Kostmann syndrome), cyclic neutropenia, leukocyte adhesion defects, Chediak–Higashi syndrome, etc. Examples of acquired immunosuppression include HIV/AIDs and medication-induced immunosuppression seen in transplant patients, as well as children undergoing chemotherapy.

The epidemiology of primary immune deficiency diseases varies and depends on the geographic region, ethnicity, race, and gender. In the United States, it is estimated that 1:2000 children have a primary immune deficiency condition.

Children with immune deficiency are more susceptible to bacterial, viral, and opportunistic fungal infections. Oftentimes, these infections can have a presentation that is atypical and occasionally severe. In addition, the oral lesions can take longer to resolve. Early detection and aggressive treatment of oral soft tissue infections are essential in children with suppressed immune systems or an immunodeficiency disorder. Cultures can be utilized in many cases to help identify the infectious agent, thus ensuring appropriate treatment.

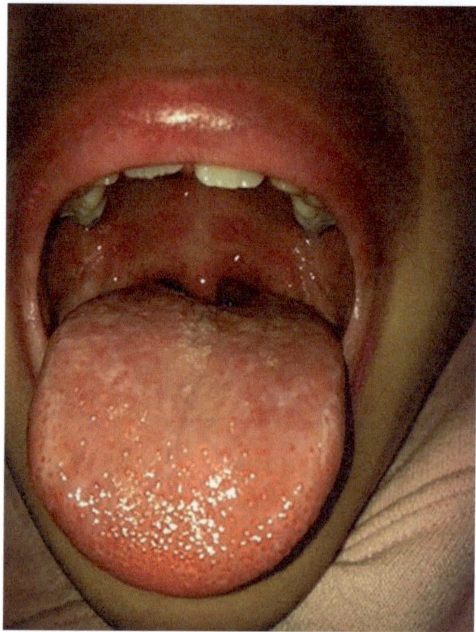

Fig. 2.9 Lichenoid mucositis in graft versus host disease. 8-year old immunosuppressed, renal transplant female recipient who presented with multiple punctate ulcers of the posterior soft palate and white lichenoid lesions on the dorsal tongue

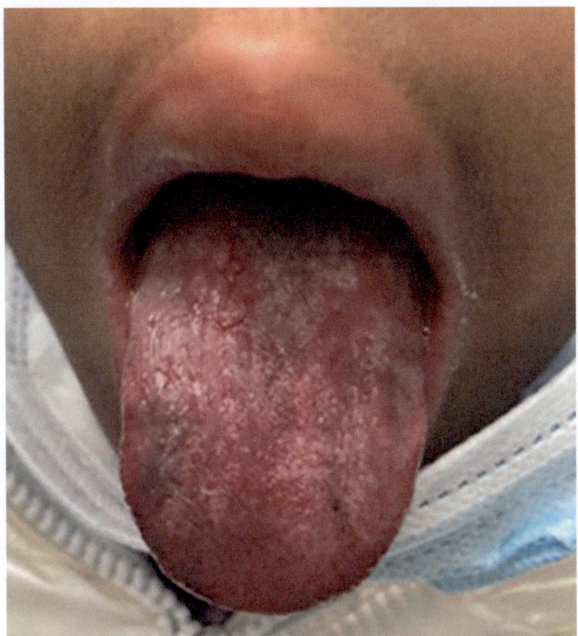

Fig. 2.10 *Candidiasis* of tongue in a 7-year-old patient status post-stem cell transplant for sickle cell anemia and chronic graft versus host disease. Pigmentations of the tongue are also seen. The pigmentations could be physiological or post-inflammatory

HIV/AIDs

According to the World Health Organization, in 2021, an estimated 1.7 million children were living with HIV.

Oral Lesions Associated with HIV/AIDs
Candidiasis
HIV-related gingivitis
Necrotizing ulcerative gingivitis/periodontitis/stomatitis
Kaposi sarcoma
Oral hairy leukoplakia
Recurrent ulcers
Warts
Parotid gland enlargement

Oral lesions most often occur when a patient's CD4 count is less than 200 cells/mm^3. It is important to note that the incidence of HIV-related salivary gland disease, HPV-associated lesions, and recurrent ulcerations have increased incidence in adult patients taking HAART therapy. It is not yet clear if the incidence is increased for children receiving HAART therapy.

Clinical Note

Prior to treating an immunocompromised child, it is important to review the results of a current complete blood cell count with white cell differential. Consultation with the child's pediatrician or medical specialist to discuss the child's oral health and any significant clinical findings is recommended.

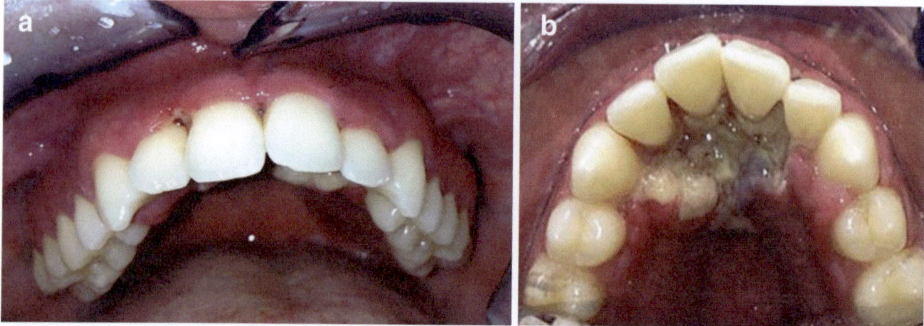

Fig. 2.11 (**a, b**) Necrotizing ulcerative stomatitis. Punched out and necrotic appearance of facial gingiva (**a**) and a large irregular ulcer with necrotic tissue of the anterior palatal gingiva extending to the hard palate (**b**) in an HIV-positive young adult

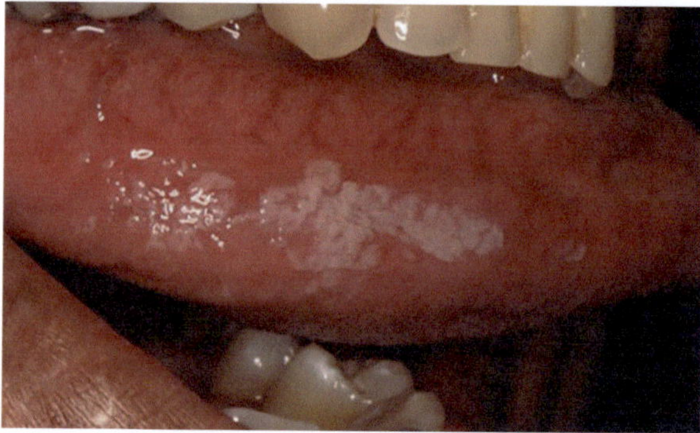

Fig. 2.12 Oral hairy leukoplakia. Non-removable white patch of the lateral tongue in an HIV-positive patient. Patient is an adult

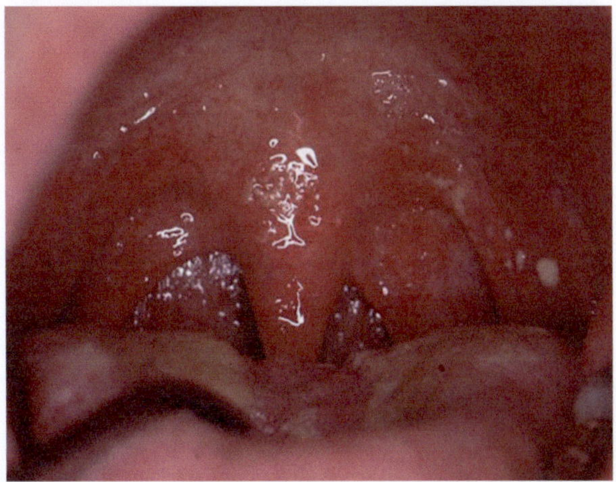

Fig. 2.13 Oro-pharyngeal candidiasis. Removable white plaques from the posterior soft palate. Median rhomboid glossitis is also present

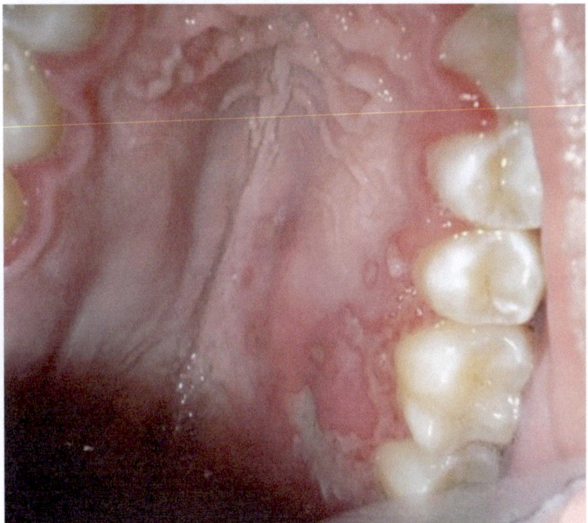

Fig. 2.14 Recurrent intraoral herpetic infection. Multiple ulcerations limited to left palatal gingiva and left side of the palate

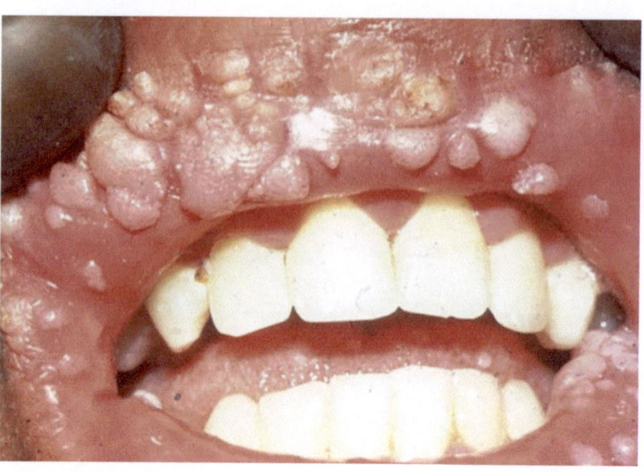

Fig. 2.15 HIV-associated oral papillomas. Multiple exophytic papillomatous lesions of the upper and lower lip mucosa

2.4   Oral Manifestations of Habits and Abuse

Physical Abuse
Injuries to the head and neck occur in over 50% of child abuse cases. A careful and thorough extraoral and intraoral examination must be performed. Intraoral findings of physical abuse include mucosal ulcers, lacerations, ecchymosis, and burns of the tongue, lips, buccal mucosa, hard and soft palate, gingiva, alveolar mucosa, and frenum. Such injuries can be sustained by eating utensils or bottles during forced feedings, or from the forced ingestion of scalding hot foods, liquids, or caustic substances. Lacerations of the gingiva, lip, and frenum can also be caused by extraoral trauma from the hands of the abuser. Facial bruises, injuries to the ears, fractured or avulsed teeth, and jaw or zygomatic fractures are also findings in cases of physical abuse. Injuries observed in exposed skin of the extremities including scars, bruises, cigarette burns, and bite marks are also highly indicative of physical abuse.

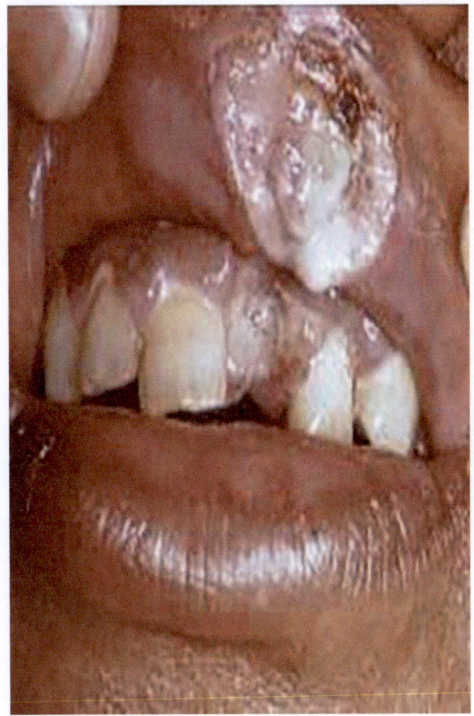

Fig. 2.16 Physical abuse. Avulsed central incisor and ulcerated upper lip as a result of inflicted trauma

Accidental injuries to the mouth are not uncommon in children. Therefore, it is critical to distinguish accidental injuries from abuse. Multiple injuries, injuries in different stages of healing, or doubtful history of how the injury occurred should arouse a suspicion of abuse.

Child Neglect

Oral findings in children suffering from neglect include rampant tooth decay, gingivitis, and generalized poor oral health. These children may also appear unkempt and show signs of nutritional deficiencies.

Dental neglect is a form of child abuse. The American Academy of Pediatric Dentistry defines dental neglect as a "willful failure of parent or guardian to seek and follow through with treatment necessary to ensure a level of oral health essential for adequate function and freedom from pain and infection." Some parents/guardians fail to seek dental care for their children because they are not educated on the importance of childhood dental health. Therefore, the clinician must attempt to educate the parents/guardian. If access to care or finances are the issue, clinicians should provide information on available mechanisms for appropriate evaluation and treatment.

Sexual Abuse

Oral findings seen in children suffering sexual abuse include oral and perioral gonorrhea, oral condyloma, and injury or petechiae of the palate.

Note: Palatal petechiae are not pathognomonic of sexual abuse. Palatal petechiae can occur as a result of heavy coughing, and with various viral and bacterial infections such as herpangina and strep throat.

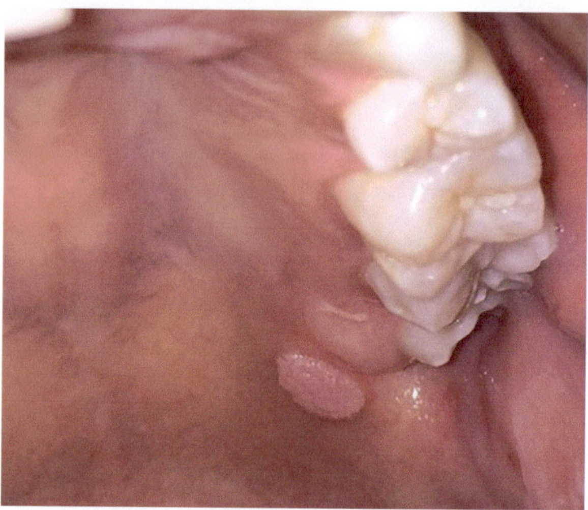

Fig. 2.17 Oral Condyloma. Pale pink cauliflower-like growth of soft palate

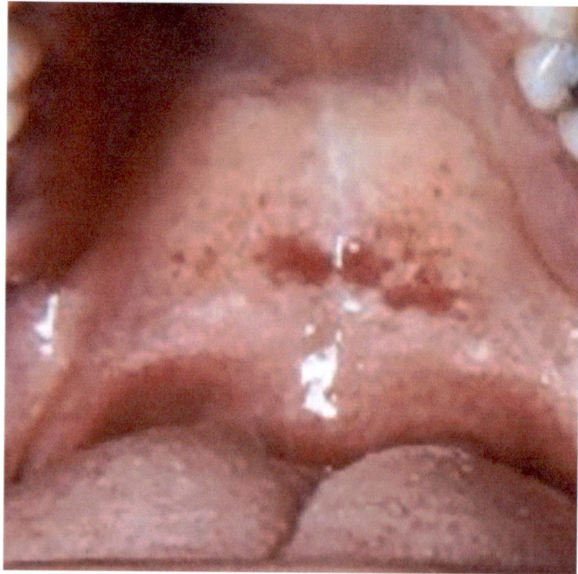

Fig. 2.18 Petechiae. Petechial hemorrhage of the soft palate

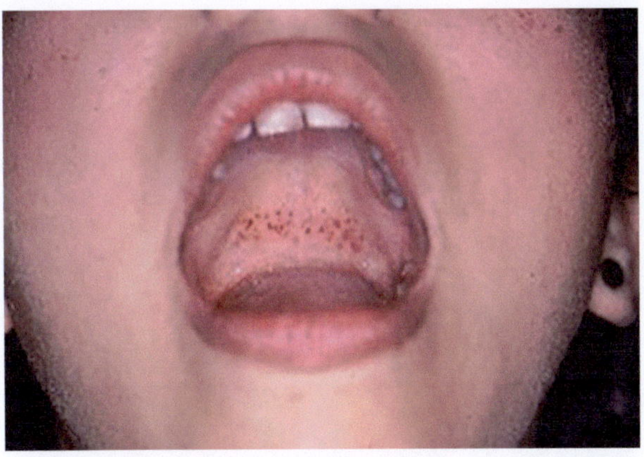

Fig. 2.19 Petechiae. Petechial hemorrhage of the soft palate

All cases of the suspected physical/sexual abuse or child neglect must be reported to child protective services and/or law enforcement agencies including state departments of health for investigation

Eating Disorders

Eating disorders often develop during adolescence. However, they can start in childhood. The prevalence of eating disorders in young children has been growing. Girls are more frequently affected. Eating disorders include anorexia nervosa, bulimia nervosa, and binge eating. Avoidant/Restrictive Food Intake Disorder is a type of eating disturbance in which a sufferer fails to meet an adequate body weight but does not fit in the diagnostic criteria for anorexia or bulimia.

Children with eating disorders often exhibit signs of malnutrition. Mucosal findings include mucosal atrophy, glossitis, and gingivitis resulting from vitamin deficiencies. Children with bulimia frequently show erythema and/or petechiae of the soft palate as a result of injury from purging, hyperkeratosis, and scarring of the dorsal aspects of the fingers and hands (Russell sign) caused by repeated trauma to the finger/hand used to induce gaging/vomiting. Demineralization and loss of tooth enamel result from recurrent vomiting followed by toothbrushing in the presence of gastric acid. Bilateral persistent enlargement of the parotid glands, referred to as sialadenosis, is another sign.

Eating disorders in children and teens can lead to a host of serious physical problems, including organ damage, heart arrhythmias, and even death. In addition, eating disorders are often associated with psychiatric problems. It is crucial that eating disorders are diagnosed and treated early. If an eating disorder is suspected in a child, the findings should be disclosed to the patient's pediatrician.

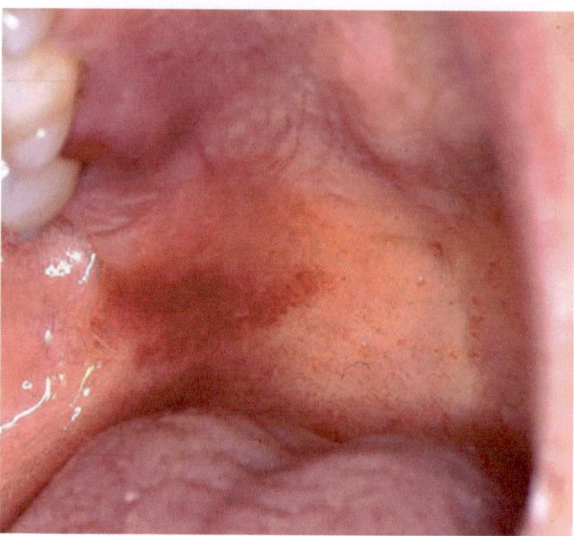

Fig. 2.20 Ecchymosis of the soft palate caused by the patient's fingers to induce vomiting

Smoking Approximately 4.5 million US teenagers smoke. According to the US Surgeon General, almost all tobacco use begins during youth and young adulthood. Children's addiction to nicotine can come from cigarette smoking, smokeless tobacco (snuff, chew), cigars, hookahs (water pipes), and vaping (e-cigarettes). The oral manifestations in teens and adolescents are the same as those seen in adults and can include leukoplakias, erythroplakias, brown hairy tongue, nicotine stomatitis, tobacco pouch keratosis (in cases of smokeless tobacco), oral submucosal fibrosis (in cases of betel quid), and squamous cell carcinoma.

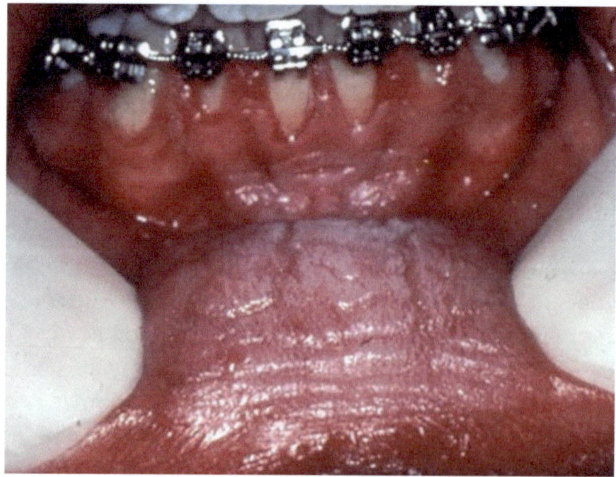

Fig. 2.21 Tobacco pouch keratosis. Teenaged snuff user. White patch with and corrugations at site of snuff placement. Also note the localized gingival recession on the adjacent teeth

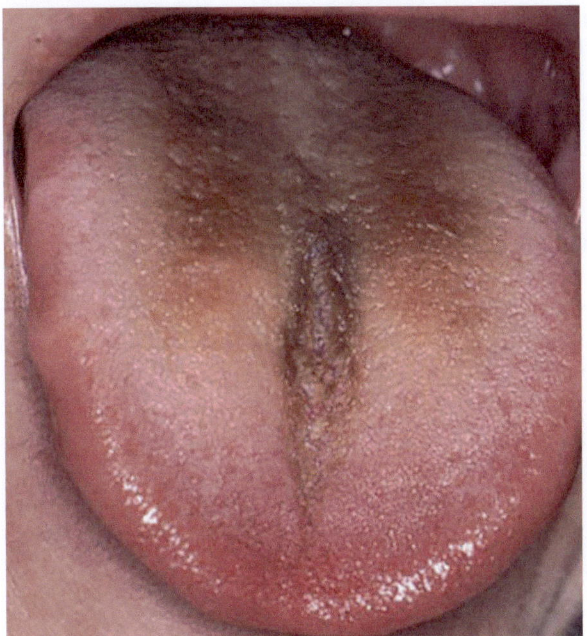

Fig. 2.22 Brown coated/hairy tongue. Diffuse light brown discoloration of the dorsal tongue

Illicit Drug Use

As it is the case with nicotine, illicit drug use often begins during youth and young adulthood. Oral manifestations vary depending on the type of drug that is abused and include a rapid increase in dental caries (especially on the labial and buccal cervical third of the teeth), gingival recession, dental erosion, bruxism, xerostomia, leukoplakias, and erythroplakias. Allergic thrombocytopenia, caused by quinine in adulterated heroin, can manifest with ecchymosis of the oral mucosa. Erythema/mucosal burns can result from smoked crack cocaine.

Drug abusers often develop nutritional deficiencies characterized by oral manifestations described above (See Sect. 2.2).

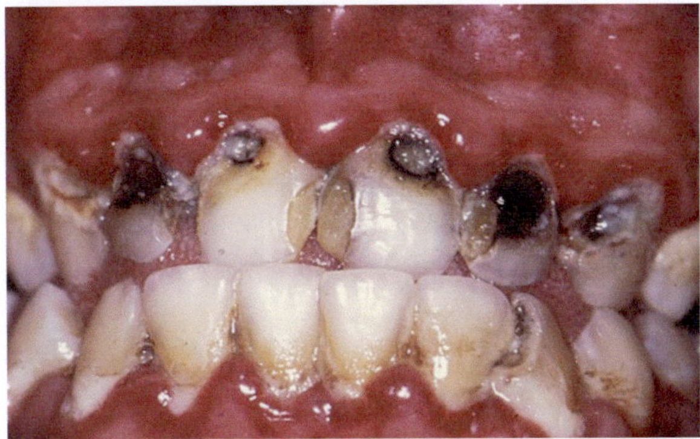

Fig. 2.23 Poor oral hygiene characterized by *gingivitis and rampant tooth decay*

2.5 Oral Soft Tissue Manifestations of Hematologic Disorders

Hematologic disorders can exhibit non-specific, as well as, pathognomonic oral manifestations.

2.5.1 White Blood Cell Disorders

Cyclic Neutropenia (Cyclic Hematopoiesis) Cyclic neutropenia most commonly presents in infants and children. Patients typically experience recurring episodes of fever, ear infections, sore throat, oral ulcerations, and skin infections. These manifestations correspond with transient neutropenia that occurs at cyclical intervals of 15–35 days (most commonly 21 days). Oral manifestations of cyclic neutropenia include recurrent aphthous stomatitis, recurrent gingivitis, and periodontitis. Oral lesions occur during the nadir and improve or resolve as the neutrophil count improves.

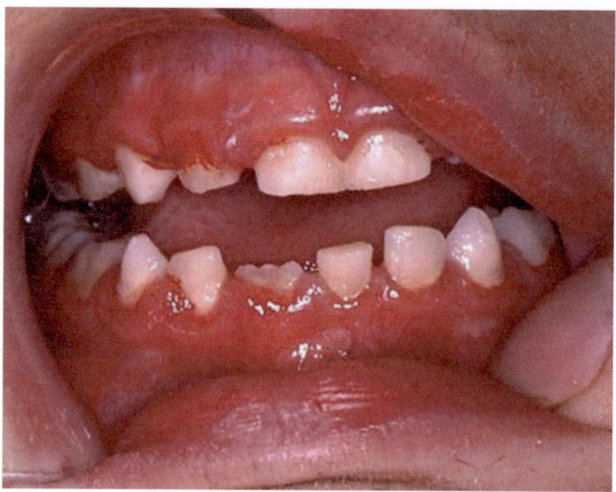

Fig. 2.24 Gingivitis. Inflamed gingiva in a child with *cyclic neutropenia*

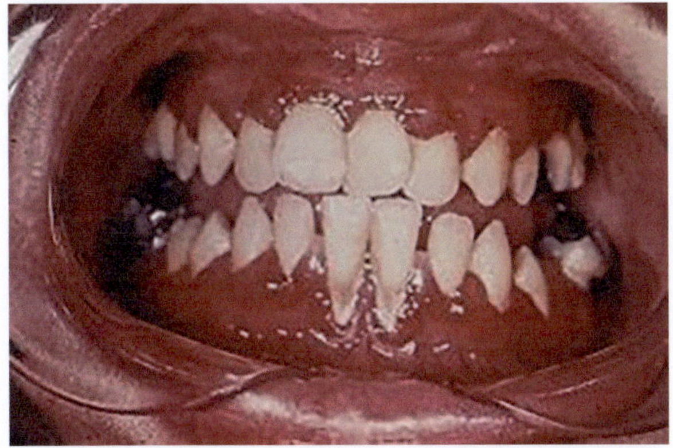

Fig. 2.25 Gingivitis and marked localized recession in an adolescent with *cyclic neutropenia*

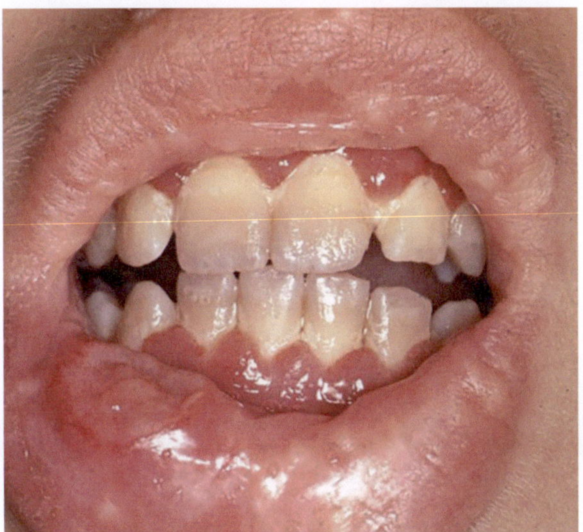

Fig. 2.26 Inflamed gingiva and a major aphthous ulceration of the lower lip mucosa

Leukemia Clinical manifestations of leukemia result from loss of normal leukocyte function, suppression of hematopoietic cell lines, or direct infiltration of leukemic cells into tissues. Systemic signs and symptoms include fatigue, anemia, lymphadenopathy, recurrent infection, bone and abdominal pain, bleeding, and purpura. Oral manifestations include mucosal, gingival bleeding and mucosal petechiae, and oral ulcerations. Patients are also susceptible to bacterial, fungal, and viral oral infections, that can be severe, as a consequence of immunosuppression. A leukemic infiltrate of the gingiva presents as swollen, erythematous, and friable gingiva.

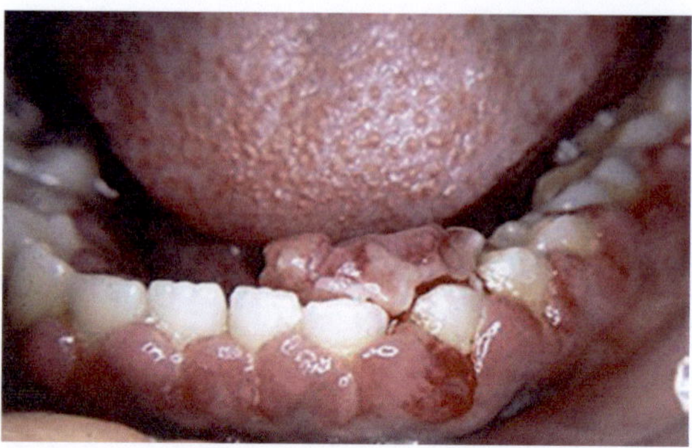

Fig. 2.27 *Leukemic infiltrate* of the mandibular gingiva. Note the spontaneous bleeding and puffiness (arrow)

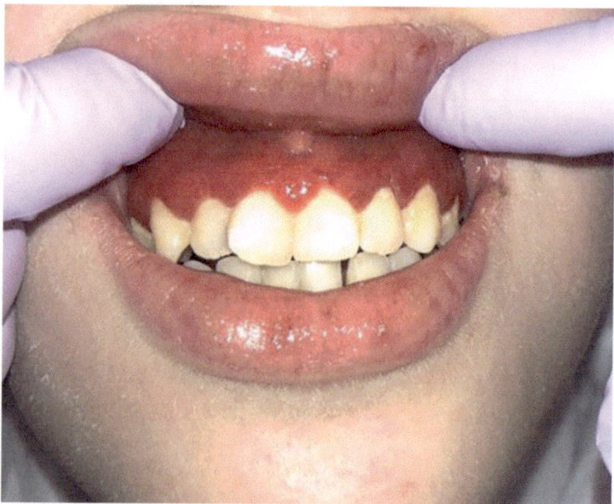

Fig. 2.28 Leukemic infiltrate. Erythema and swelling of the maxillary gingiva in a teenage patient with recently diagnosed acute lymphocytic leukemia

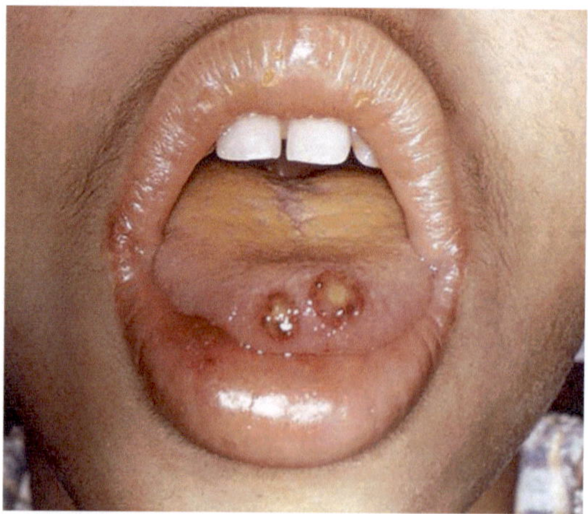

Fig. 2.29 Multiple painful ulcers on the anterior dorsal tongue and right lower lip in an adolescent with leukemia

Lymphomas Clinical manifestations of lymphoma are variable and can include painless lymphadenopathy, hepatosplenomegaly, secondary infections, fever, night sweats, and weight loss. Lymphoma can manifest in the oral cavity as a tonsillar mass or as a diffuse, boggy mass, particularly of the gingiva or palate with or without secondary surface ulceration.

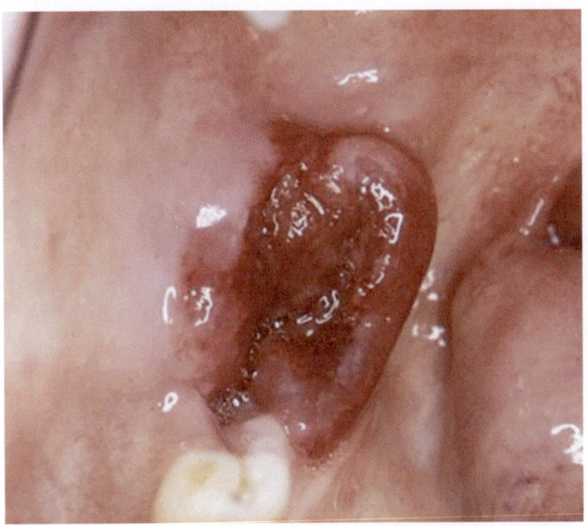

Fig. 2.30 B-cell non-Hodgkin's lymphoma. Ulcerated, erythematous, non-painful, soft tissue mass of the retromolar region

Burkitt lymphoma is an aggressive pediatric lymphoma that is commonly associated with oral manifestations. The African or endemic type often occurs in the jaw and presents as a rapidly expanding mass causing bone and adjacent soft tissue destruction, resulting in painful loosening of the teeth.

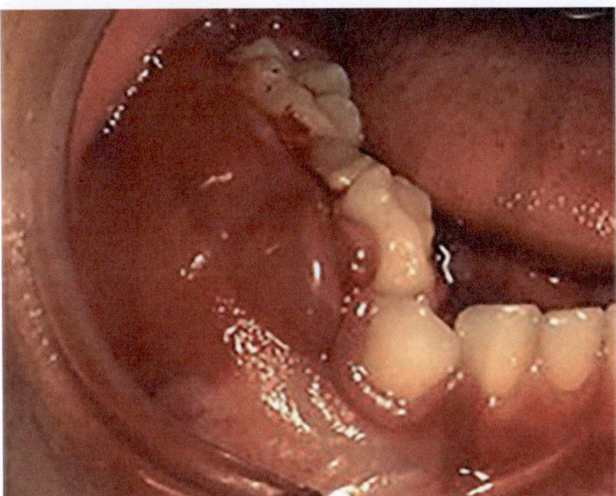

Fig. 2.31 Burkitt lymphoma. Dusky red/erythematous, soft tissue mass of the posterior mandible with underlying bone destruction

Langerhans' Cell Histiocytosis It is characterized by a spectrum of clinical manifestations depending on the site and extent of organ involvement. It may be present as an isolated bone lesion or as a progressive systemic disease. 10–20% of patients have lytic lesions of the maxilla or mandible with ulceration of the overlying mucosa and gingival inflammation. Ulceration of the oral mucosa in the absence of underlying bone lesions can also occur but this presentation is rare.

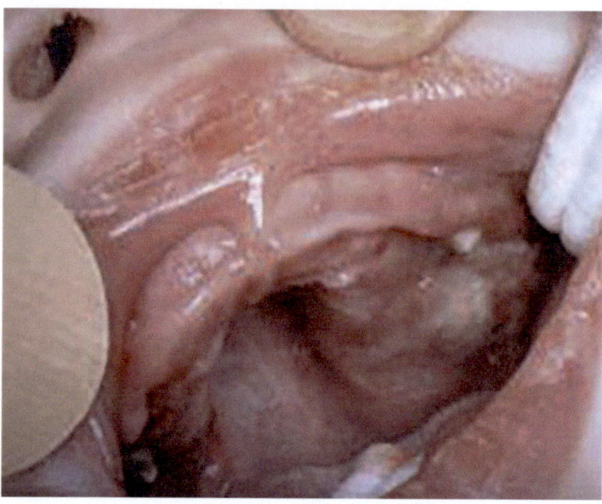

Fig. 2.32 *Langerhans' cell histiocytosis* manifesting as a ulcerated swelling involving the maxillary alveolus and palate in an infant

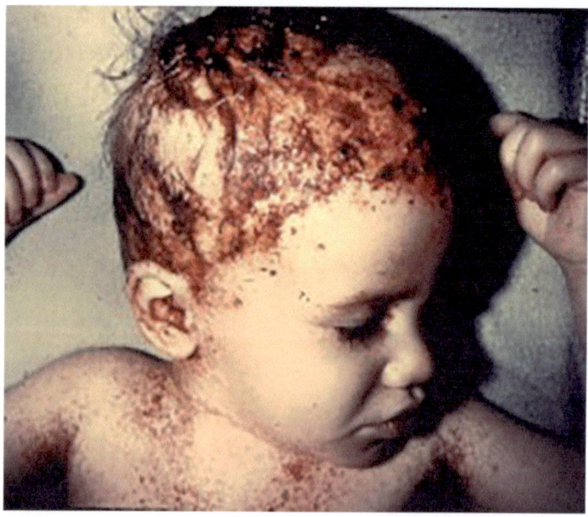

Fig. 2.33 *Langerhans' cell histiocytosis* manifesting as a wide-spread cutaneous rash ulcerated swelling involving the maxillary alveolus and palate in an infant

2.5.2   Red Blood Cell Disorders

Anemia   Regardless of the cause, anemia may result in gingival and/or mucosal pallor, glossitis, glossodynia, and stomatitis. Oral findings may be the initial presentation of anemia due to iron, folate, or vitamin B12 deficiencies.

Sickle Cell Disease   The most common oral mucosal manifestations are gingival/mucosal pallor or jaundice of the palate, buccal mucosa, and gingiva due to hemolysis.

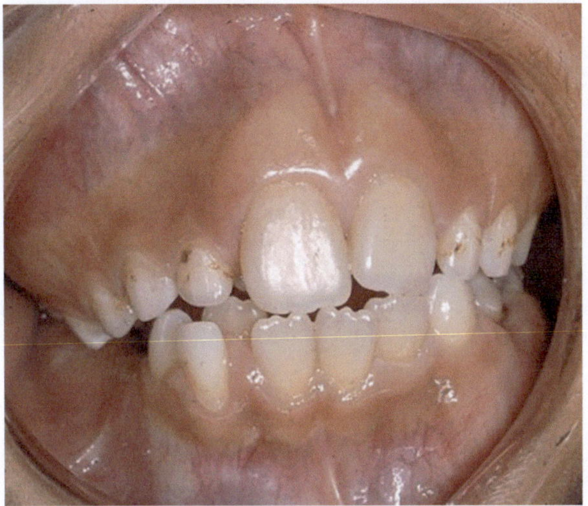

Fig. 2.34   Gingival and vestibular mucosa pallor in child with sickle cell anemia

Hemochromatosis   The primary oral manifestation of hereditary hemochromatosis, or any state of iron overload, is blue-gray to brown hyperpigmentation that most commonly affects the palate, buccal mucosa, and gingiva.

2.5.3   Platelet Disorders

Thrombocytopenia

Regardless of the cause, platelet disorders typically manifest as petechiae, purpuras, and/or bleeding of the oral mucosa. Gingival bleeding, either spontaneous or in response to minor trauma (i.e., toothbrushing and flossing), is often the first sign of thrombocytopenia.

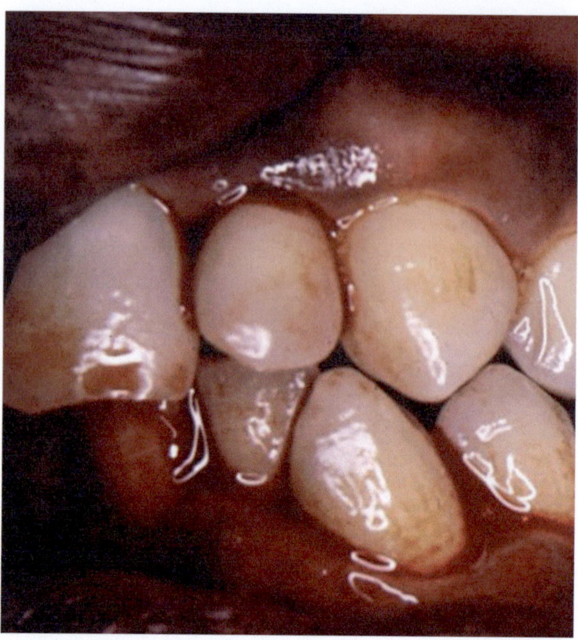

Fig. 2.35 Spontaneous gingival bleeding in a patient with significant thrombocytopenia

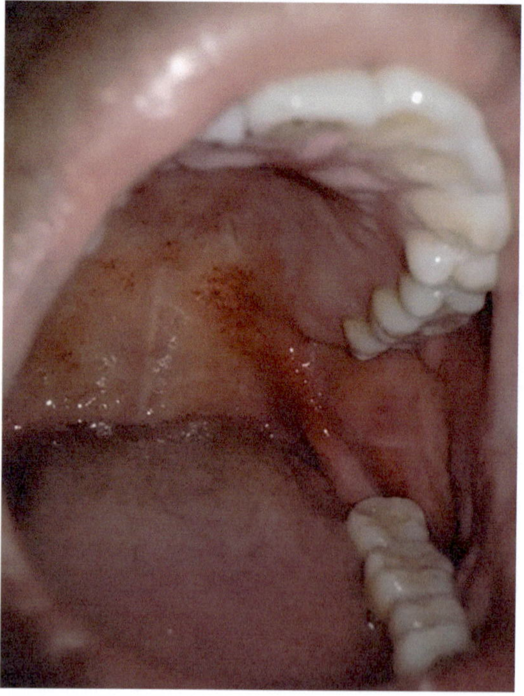

Fig. 2.36 Petechial hemorrhage of the soft palate occurring in a thrombocytopenic patient

Part III

Sample Cases

Case 1

Patient is a 10-year-old female. Her mom brought her in for evaluation of "'black spots on tongue," which were first noticed that morning. The patient has no known medical problems and appears in good health. She is recovering from a recent "stomach bug." (Photo courtesy of Dr. Andrea Mann).

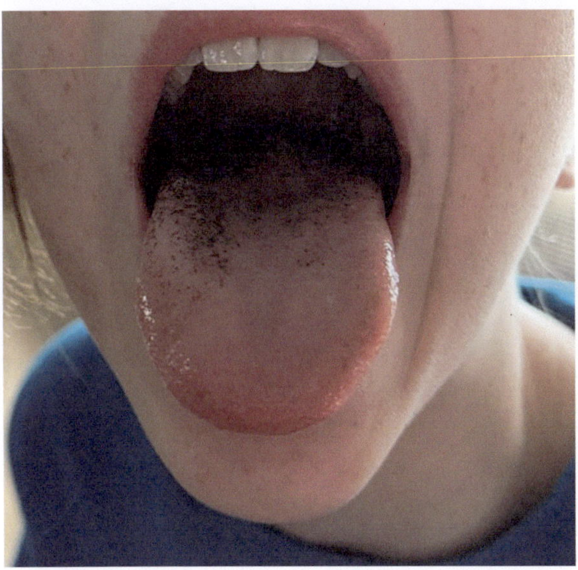

The presentation is characteristic of brown/black coated tongue. Upon questioning the parent, it was confirmed that the child had been given Pepto-Bismol for a "stomach bug." The bismuth in Pepto-Bismol reacts with trace amounts of sulfur in the saliva resulting in a black stain. The stain is harmless and will fade. Brushing the tongue can speed up the process. Confirmation of the clinical diagnosis can be made by follow-up. The pigmentation should disappear within 14 days barring exposure to bismuth.

Case 2
A healthy 11-year-old male presents for a hygiene appointment. During examination you notice the gingival lesion shown below. The lesion is located on the buccal surface of the patient's primary molar, which has a stainless steel crown. The child is asymptomatic. Bitewing and periapical radiographs of the tooth are unremarkable (Photo courtesy of Dr. Andrea Mann).

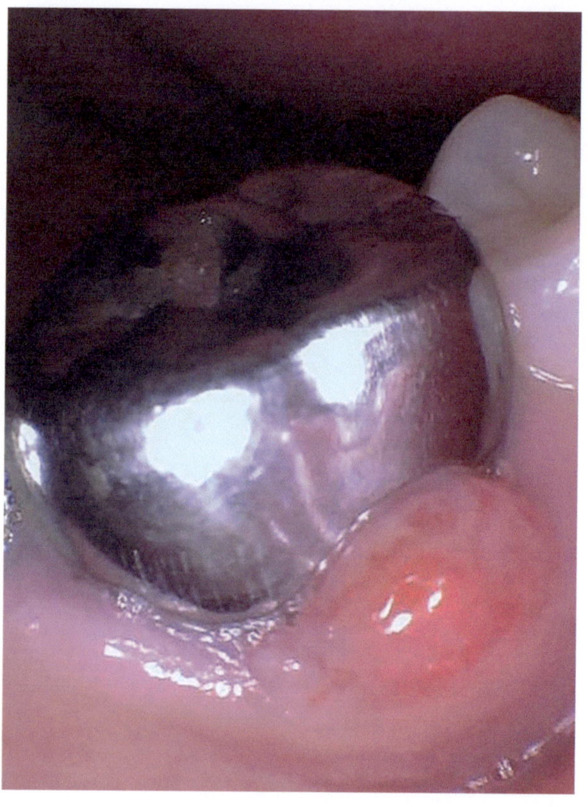

As stated in the section on gingival lesions, whenever a patient presents with gingival swelling, the clinician should evaluate the underlying bone with a radiograph. The differential diagnosis for this focal gingival nodule with normal radiographic findings include pyogenic granuloma, peripheral ossifying fibroma, fibroma that is secondarily inflamed, and peripheral giant cell granuloma (less likely). Of the entities listed pyogenic granuloma is favored. Peripheral giant cell granuloma is less likely based on the age of the patient. Since the tooth has a stainless steel crown, excess cement at the margin or lack of proper home hygiene are potential irritants that could lead to a pyogenic granuloma. Parulis is also less likely due to the location of the lesion at the attached and marginal gingiva. Parulides occur on the gingiva at the level of the tooth root apex. Also, it is stated in the history that the radiographic examination was unremarkable. The definitive diagnosis for this gingival nodule requires surgical excision followed by histopathologic examination. The final diagnosis, in this case, was pyogenic granuloma.

Case 3

A 10-year-old female presents with the following complaint: "My cheek hurts really bad when I eat." On clinical examination, you discover a well-defined, irregularly shaped ulceration on the right buccal mucosa. The ulcer is soft to palpation. No other lesions are present. Upon questioning, the patient states that she first noticed pain 3 days ago when she woke up in the morning. The child appears in good health and a review of her medical history is unremarkable (Photo courtesy of Dr. Andrea Mann).

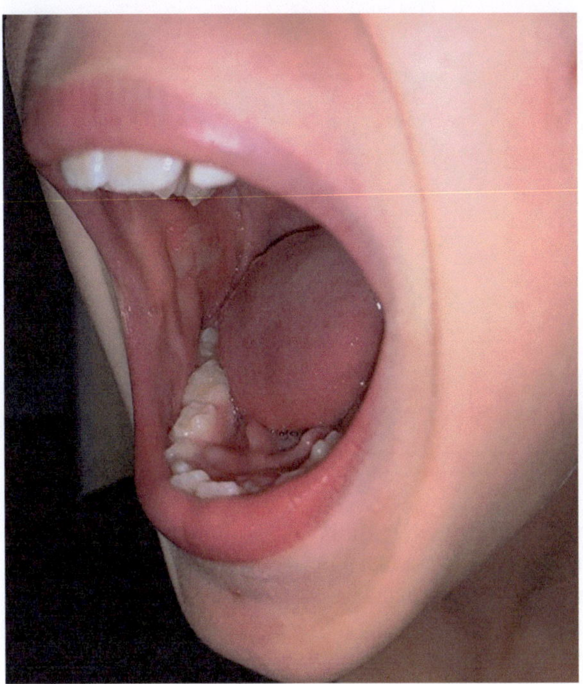

Although the patient does not recall biting her cheek, the clinical presentation is consistent with a traumatic ulcer. Note the sharp appearance of the maxillary molar cusps. The clinical diagnosis can be confirmed by smoothing the sharp cusps and having the patient return for follow-up in 2 weeks. Triamcinolone in Orabase® can provide some symptomatic relief. If the lesion fails to heal in 2 weeks after addressing potential causes (i.e., sharp cusps) biopsy is recommended. When the patient returned for follow-up 7 days later, the lesion was completely healed.

Case 4

A healthy 2-year old is brought in for his initial dental visit. You notice a brown pigmented lesion of the attached gingiva with well-defined borders measuring about 4 × 2 mm. The child's parents said that the lesion was noticed while brushing the baby's teeth a few months ago (Photo courtesy of Dr. Andrea Mann).

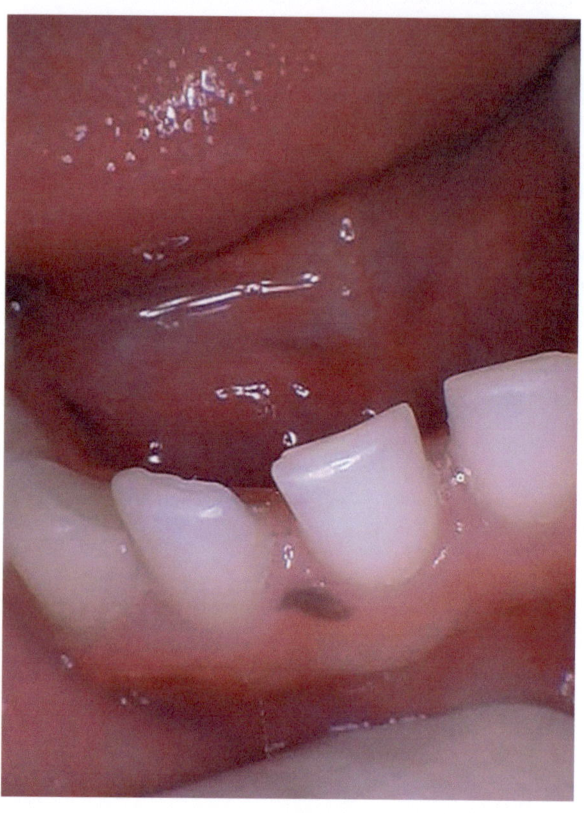

The differential diagnosis for this focal pigmented lesion in a young child includes melanotic macule or melanocytic nevus (i.e., blue nevus). An amalgam tattoo can be excluded based on the patient's age and history. Melanoma is extremely unlikely given the patient's age and clinical presentation (i.e., smooth borders and uniform color). Ethnic/racial pigmentation would not be focal and as well-defined. A definitive diagnosis requires a biopsy. However, since the clinical presentation appears benign an acceptable conservative approach could be to monitor the lesion and reserve biopsy should the lesion demonstrate any significant changes in size, color, and/or surface quality.

Case 5

The parents of a healthy one-year brought in their infant for evaluation after noticing something on the child's roof of mouth. Clinical examination revealed a round tan, smooth, slightly raised lesion on the palate (Photographs courtesy of Dr. Mackenzie Tappe).

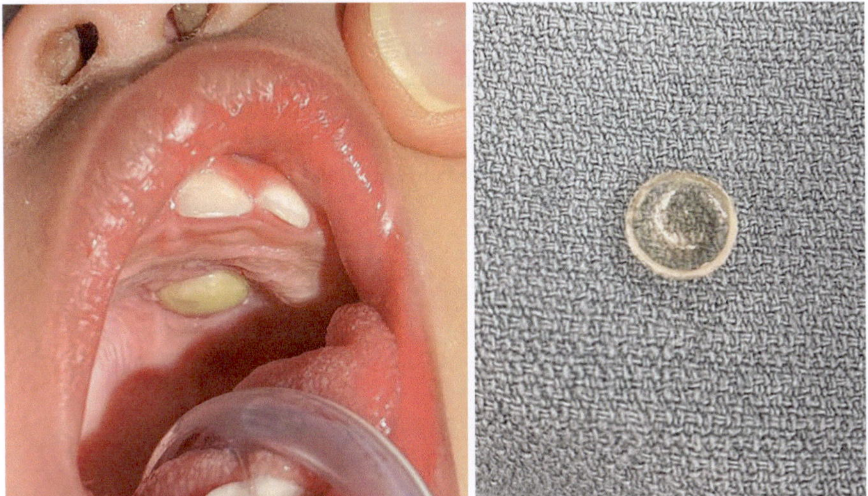

The tan-yellow color could be suggestive of an ulcer, because the lesion looked raised differential would include soft tissue tumor with surface ulceration. Palpation is an essential component of clinical examination. On palpation, the area of concern felt hard. The "lesion" was a foreign body that was stuck to the palate. This was an unusual case.

Case 6

A 7-year-old child was brought in for evaluation of a "growth" on his upper lip. The child was asymptomatic and in good health. As per the child's mother, the growth was present for about 3 months. Clinical examination revealed the lesion to be pedunculated with a stalk-like attachment to the lip. No other lesions were present on intraoral examination.

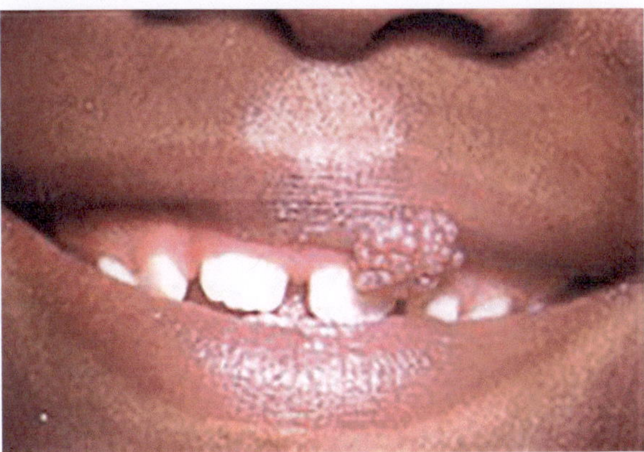

The clinical presentation is characteristic of an HPV-related lesion. The differential includes a squamous papilloma or verruca vulgaris. If the child had any cutaneous warts on his fingers, verruca vulgaris would be favored. Condyloma acuminatum could be considered. The upper lip is a common site for oral condyloma acuminatum, however, most occur as multiple lesions and the lesions are more often sessile rather than pedunculated. Multifocal Viral Epithelial Hyperplasia (Heck's disease) is not likely due to the isolated presentation. Treatment is surgical excision. Microscopic examination confirmed the clinical diagnosis of squamous papilloma. Recurrence is possible but unlikely.

Case 7
The parents of a healthy 18 months old noticed the cutaneous lesions depicted below. The child had a low-grade fever, loss of appetite, and experienced crankiness. Photos courtesy of Dr. Jill White, Veteran Affairs Hospital, San Francisco CA

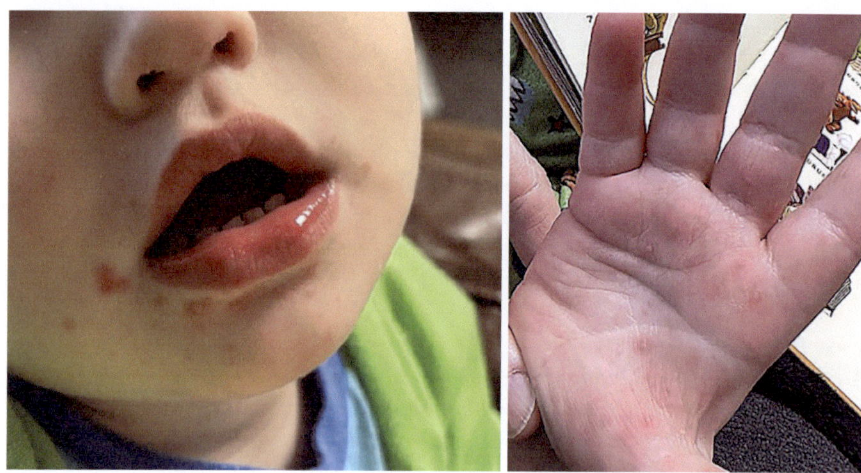

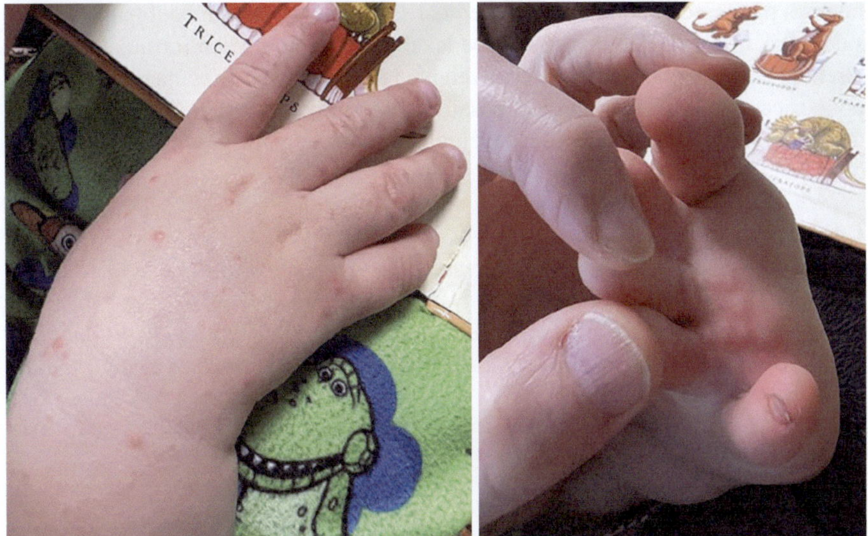

This child presented with characteristic signs and symptoms of hand, foot and mouth disease. Intraoral ulcers and a rash or blisters on the legs and buttocks are also common. The diagnosis was clinical and the patient was treated with palliative care and fully recovered 1 week later.

Case 8

An adolescent male presented for evaluation of growth of his lower lip. Although it was not painful, he was concerned about the appearance and reported that it bled when he touched it. According to the patient—he bit his lip in that spot a few months ago and developed a bump that has progressively gotten bigger. Clinical exam did not reveal any other oral or perioral lesions.

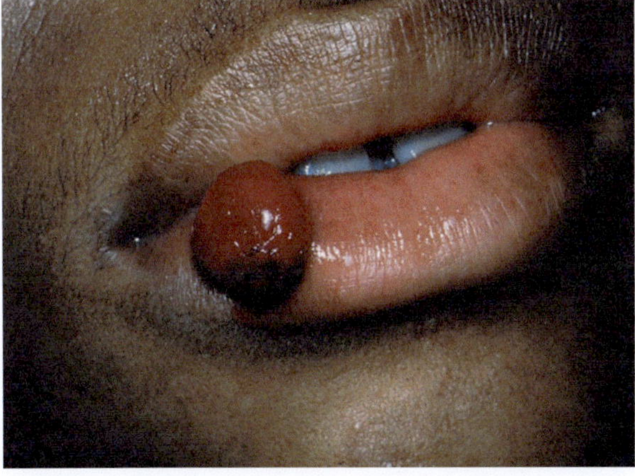

The development of a soft tissue mass of the lower lip after reported trauma might initially suggest a mucocele. However, the clinical appearance and report of bleeding when manipulated are not typical of mucoceles. The clinical presentation favors a pyogenic granuloma. An ulcerated soft tissue neoplasm could also be considered. A history of trauma should be taken into account when formulating a differential diagnosis but should not be weighted too heavily since some patients might not be accurate historians and it is possible that a traumatic event could be incidental. In this case, trauma led to the development of a pyogenic granuloma which was confirmed by excisional biopsy.

Case 9

A 9-year old presents for a routine hygiene appointment with the ulcerated lesion shown below. Upon questioning the child's parent reports it has been there for about a week. The child was complaining that it hurt a few days ago but is not bothering her now. The parent reports that she gets similar sores on her lip.

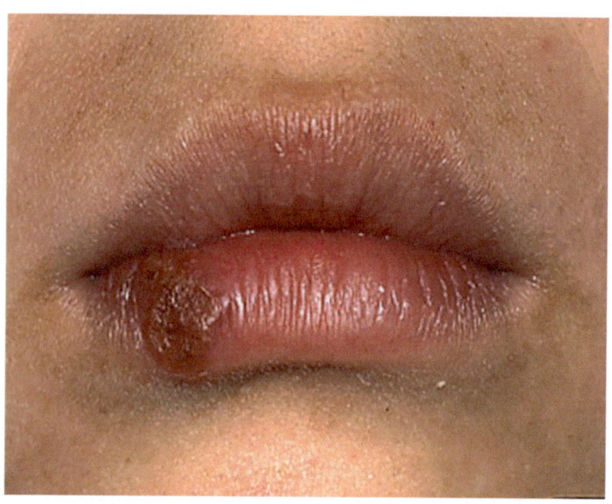

This is a classic presentation of herpes labialis, commonly referred to as a cold sore. It is caused by the herpes simplex virus. Cold sores are typically not treated in children since antiviral medications need to be started at the prodromal stage in order to be most effective. If taken during an outbreak antiviral medication can reduce symptoms and shorten the duration only by a day or two. Should an antiviral medication be prescribed, oral acyclovir is the antiviral most often used in children. Oral acyclovir does not have any age-specified indications according to the FDA label. Topical antiviral creams are recommended for those 12 years and older. Children should avoid touching/picking at cold sores since this can spread the virus to other parts of the body, such as fingers and eyes, as well as to other children. Children should also therefore be encouraged to wash their hands frequently. Since the sores remain highly contagious until the skin completely heals, it is best to defer the patient's dental appointment.

Case 10

A 16-year old presents with a fluctuant polypoid mass, with a slight bluish appearance. He reports that it sometimes gets larger, sometimes smaller but it never goes away. It is not painful but is annoying since he can feel it there.

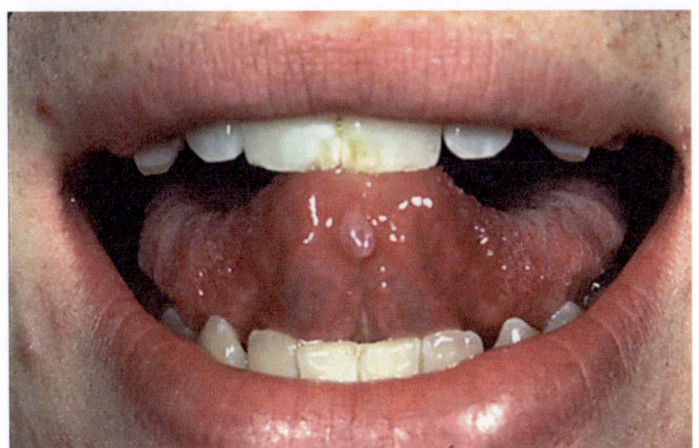

The clinical presentation is consistent with a mucocele. Other considerations might include a pyogenic granuloma or fibroma. Mucocele's of the ventral tongue are caused by the anterior lingual salivary glands (glands of Blandin–Nuhn). These are mixed mucous and serous glands that are embedded within the musculature of anterior tongue ventrum. In order to avoid recurrence, mucoceles of the glands of Blandin and Nuhn should be removed up to the muscle plane, together with the small glands found in the surgical field.

References

Allen CM, Blozis GG. Oral mucosal reactions to cinnamon-flavored chewing gum. J Am Dent Assoc. 1988;116:664–7.

American Academy of Pediatric Dentistry. Clinical guideline on oral and dental aspects of child abuse and neglect. Pediatr Dent. 2004;26(7 Suppl):63–6.

BaniHani A, Nazzal H, Webb L, Toumba KJ, Fabbroni G. An unusual presentation of erythema multiforme in a paediatric patient. Eur Arch Paediatr Dent. 2015;16(3):297–302.

Blokzijl ML. Human immunodeficiency virus infection in childhood. Ann Trop Paediatr. 1988;8(1):1–17.

Carlson ER, Ord RA. Benign pediatric salivary gland lesions. Oral Maxillofac Surg Clin North Am. 2016;28(1):67–81.

Cavalcante RB, Turatti E, Daniel AP, de Alencar GF, Chen Z. Retrospective review of oral and maxillofacial pathology in a Brazilian paediatric population. Eur Arch Paediatr Dent. 2016;17(2):115–22.

Darling MR, Daley TD, Wilson A, Wysocki GP. Juvenile spongiotic gingivitis. J Periodontol. 2007;78:1235–40.

daSilva FC, Piazzetta CM, Torres-Pereira CC, Schussel JL, Amenábar JM. Gingival proliferative lesions in children and adolescents in Brazil: a 15-year-period cross-sectional study. J Indian Soc Periodontol. 2016;20(1):63–6.

Dunlap CL, Vincent SK, Barker BF. Allergic reaction to orthodontic wire: report of case. J Am Dent Assoc. 1989;118(4):449–50.

Edwards RM, Chapman T, Horn DL, Paladin AM, Iyer RS. Imaging of pediatric floor of mouth lesions. Pediatr Radiol. 2013;43(5):523–35.

Hartman-Adams H, Banvard C, Juckett G. Impetigo: diagnosis and treatment. Am Fam Physician. 2014;90(4):229–35.

Joshi SR, Pendyala GS, Choudhari S, Kalburge J. Mucocele of the glands of blandin-nuhn in children: a clinical, histopathologic, and retrospective study. N Am J Med Sci. 2012;4(9):379–83.

Koutlas IG, Anbinder AL, Alshagroud R, Rodrigues Cavalcante AS, Al Kindi M, Crenshaw MM, Sapp JC, Kondolf H, Lindhurst MJ, Dudley JN, Johnston JJ, Ryan E, Rafferty K, Ganguly A, Biesecker LG. Orofacial overgrowth with peripheral nerve enlargement and perineuriomatous pseudo-onion bulb proliferations is part of the *PIK3CA*-related overgrowth spectrum. HGG Adv. 2020;1(1):100009.

Krzywicka B, Herman K, Kowalczyk-Zając M, Pytrus T. Celiac disease and its impact on the oral health status - review of the literature. Adv Clin Exp Med. 2014;23(5):675–81.

López-Sánchez A, Guijarro Guijarro B, Hernández VG. Human repercussions of foot and mouth disease and other similar viral diseases. Med Oral. 2003;8(1):26–32.

Martínez-Escala ME, Pena MG, Paricio BB, Vallverdú RM. What is your diagnosis? Multiple cobblestone-like papules on the inner aspect of the lip. Pediatr Dermatol. 2011;28(4):457–8.

Martins-Filho PR, de Santana ST, Piva MR, da Silva HF, da Silva LC, Mascarenhas-Oliveira AC, de Souza Andrade ES. A multicenter retrospective cohort study on pediatric oral lesions. J Dent Child (Chic). 2015;82(2):84–90.

Neville BW, Damm DD, Allen CM, Chi AC. Oral and maxillofacial pathology. 4th ed. St. Louis: Elsevier Saunders; 2016.

Percinoto AC, Danelon M, Crivelini MM, Cunha RF, Percinoto C. Condyloma acuminata in the tongue and palate of a sexually abused child: a case report. BMC Res Notes. 2014;7:467.

Petel R, Ashkenazi M. Pediatric intraoral high-flow arteriovenous malformation: a diagnostic challenge. Pediatr Dent. 2014;36(5):425–8.

Plauth M, Jenss H, Meyle J. Oral manifestations of Crohn's disease. An analysis of 79 cases. J Clin Gastroenterol. 1991;13(1):29–37.

Qualia CM, Brown MR, Ryan CK, Rossi TM. Oral mucosal neuromas leading to the diagnosis of multiple endocrine neoplasia type 2B in a child with intestinal pseudo-obstruction. Gastroenterol Hepatol (N Y). 2007;3(3):208–11.

Ramazani N. Child dental neglect: a short review. Int J High Risk Behav Addict. 2014;3(4):e21861.

Roth GM, Ferguson N, Wanat KA. Segmental epidermal nevus and mucosal neuromas associated with *PIK3CA*-related overgrowth spectrum disorder. JAAD Case Rep. 2018;4(10):1080–2.

Sato M, Tanaka N, Sato T, Amagasa T. Oral and maxillofacial tumours in children: a review. Br J Oral Maxillofac Surg. 1997;35(2):92–5.

Schlosser BJ, Pirigyi M, Mirowski GW. Oral manifestations of hematologic and nutritional diseases. Otolaryngol Clin N Am. 2011;44(1):183–203.

Stojanov IJ, Woo SB. Human papillomavirus and Epstein-Barr virus associated conditions of the oral mucosa. Semin Diagn Pathol. 2015;32(1):3–11.

Tempark T, Shwayder TA. Perioral dermatitis: a review of the condition with special attention to treatment options. Am J Clin Dermatol. 2014;15(2):101–13. https://doi.org/10.1007/s40257-014-0067-7.

Tröbs RB, Mader E, Friedrich T, Bennek J. Oral tumors and tumor-like lesions in infants and children. Pediatr Surg Int. 2003;19(9-10):639–45.

Index

A
Allergic contact stomatitis, 69, 70
Allergic thrombocytopenia, 135
Amalgam tattoo, 105, 107
Anemia, 141
Angular cheilitis, 74

B
Benign migratory glossitis/geographic tongue,
    74, 75, 77
Blanching, 25
Burkitt lymphoma, 139

C
Coated tongue, 114
Condyloma acuminatum, 32, 33, 149
Congenital epulis, 95, 96

E
Eruption cyst, 91, 92
Erythema multiforme (EM), 56, 57, 59
Erythema/mucosal burns, 135
Erythroplakia, 79, 80
Ethnic/racial pigmentation, 148
Excisional biopsy, 151

F
Fibroma, 14, 16, 83, 146
Focal gingival nodule, 95

G
Gastrointestinal disease
    cobblestoning, 121
    mucogingivitis, 121
    mucosal tags/folds, 121
    persistent orofacial swelling (orofacial
        granulomatosis), 121, 122
    pyostomatitis vegetans, 119
    recurrent aphthous stomatitis-like
        ulcerations, 119
Gingival bleeding, 141
Gingival lesions, 80, 146
Gingival nodules, 3, 147

H
HAART therapy, 127
Habits and abuse
    child neglect, 131
    eating disorders, 133, 134
    illicit drug use, 135
    physical abuse, 130, 131
    sexual abuse, 132
    smoking, 134, 135
Hand-foot-and-mouth disease, 41, 42, 44
Hemangioma, 17, 20
Hematologic disorders
    platelet disorders, thrombocytopenia, 141
    red blood cell disorders
        anemia, 141
        hemochromatosis, 141
        sickle cell disease, 141
    white blood cell disorders
        Burkitt lymphoma, 139
        cyclic neutropenia (cyclic hematopoi-
            esis), 136, 137
        Langerhans' cell histiocytosis, 140
        leukemia, 137, 138
        lymphoma, 139
Hemochromatosis, 141
Hereditary gingival fibromatosis, 103

Herpangina, 39–41
Herpes labialis, 60
HIV, 127

I
Immunosuppression, 126, 127
Impetigo, 61, 62
Intraoral ulcers, 151
Iron deficiency, 124

L
Langerhans' cell histiocytosis, 140
Leukemia, 137, 138
Leukemic infiltrate, 104
Leukoplakia, 77, 79
Lip licker's dermatitis, 64
Localized juvenile spongiotic gingival
     hyperplasia, 97, 98
Lymphangiomas, 21–23
Lymphoma, 139

M
Median rhomboid glossitis, 73
Melanoma, 148
Melanotic macule (focal melanosis), 107, 109
Morsicatio buccarum and linguarum, 67
Mouth-breathing gingivitis, 99–101
Mucogingivitis, 121
Mucosal and submucosal nodules
     acute herpetic gingivostomatitis (primary
          herpes), 36, 37
     allergic contact stomatitis, 69, 70
     amalgam tattoo, 105, 107
     angular cheilitis, 74
     benign migratory glossitis/geographic
          tongue, 74, 75, 77
     clinical appearance, 3
     coated tongue, 114
     condyloma acuminatum, 32, 33
     congenital epulis, 95, 96
     differential diagnosis, 4
     eruption cyst, 91, 92
     erythema multiforme (EM), 56, 57, 59
     erythroplakia, 79, 80
     etiology, 3
     fibroma, 14, 16, 83
     fibroma, giant cell variant, 83, 84
     gingival lesions, 80
     gingival/alveolar cysts of newborn, 96, 97
     hand-foot-and-mouth disease, 41, 42, 44
     hemangioma, 17, 20
     herpangina, 39–41
     herpes labialis, 60
     impetigo, 61, 62
     leukoplakia, 77, 79
     lip licker's dermatitis, 64
     localized juvenile spongiotic gingival
          hyperplasia, 97, 98
     location, 4
     lymphangiomas, 21–23
     median rhomboid glossitis, 73
     melanotic macule (focal melanosis),
          107, 109
     morsicatio buccarum and linguarum, 67
     mouth-breathing gingivitis, 99–101
     mucosal neuromas, 25–27
     mucosal nevi, 112
     multifocal viral epithelial hyperplasia
          (Heck's disease), 33, 35
     neural lesions, 25
     oral candidiasis, 71, 72
     oral ulcers, 35
     papillary lesions, 28–35
     parulis, 93, 94
     perioral dermatitis, 63, 64
     perioral lesions, 60, 84
     peripheral giant cell granuloma, 88–90
     peripheral ossifying fibroma, 84, 86, 88
     physiologic (racial) pigmentation, 110
     pigmented lesions, 105
     plunging ranula, 10
     pyogenic granuloma, 16, 80, 82
     ranula, 7
     recurrent aphthous stomatitis, 49, 55
     recurrent intraoral herpes, 38
     salivary gland tumors, 13, 14
     soft tissue sarcomas, 27, 28
     squamous papilloma, 30, 31
     superficial chemical burn, 68, 69
     traumatic ulcer, 44, 48
     treatment, 4, 7
     vascular malformation, 25
     verruca vulgaris, 28
Mucosal manifestations
     gastrointestinal disease, 119, 121, 122
     of immunosuppression, 126, 127
     nutritional deficiencies, 123, 125
Mucosal neuromas, 25–27
Mucosal nevi, 112
Multifocal viral epithelial hyperplasia (Heck's
     disease), 33, 35, 150

N
Neural lesions, 25
Nutritional deficiencies
    cobalamin (Vitamin B12), 125
    iron deficiency, 124
    vitamin A deficiency, 125
    vitamin B2, B3, B6 and B9 deficiency, 125
    vitamin C deficiency, 125
    vitamin K, 125

O
Oral acyclovir, 152
Oral candidiasis, 71, 72
Oral lesions, 127, 136
Oral ulcers, 35

P
Palpation, 149
Papillary lesions, 28–35
Parulis, 93, 94
Perioral dermatitis, 63, 64
Perioral lesions, 60, 84
Peripheral giant cell granuloma, 88–90, 146
Peripheral ossifying fibroma, 146
Persistent orofacial swelling (orofacial
        granulomatosis), 121, 122
Physiologic (racial) pigmentation, 110
Pigmented lesions, 105
Platelet disorders, thrombocytopenia, 141
Plunging ranula, 10
Pyogenic granuloma, 16, 80, 82, 146, 151, 153
Pyostomatitis vegetans, 119

R
Ranula, 7
Recurrent aphthous stomatitis, 49, 55

Recurrent aphthous stomatitis herpeti-
        formis, 54
Recurrent intraoral herpes, 38
Red blood cell disorders
    anemia, 141
    hemochromatosis, 141
    sickle cell disease, 141

S
Salivary gland tumors, 13, 14
Sickle cell disease, 141
Soft tissue sarcomas, 27, 28
Squamous papilloma, 30,
        31, 150
Superficial chemical burn, 68, 69

T
Thrombocytopenia, 141
Topical antiviral creams, 152
Traumatic ulcer, 44, 48

V
Vascular malformation, 25
Verruca vulgaris, 28
Vitamin A deficiency, 125

W
White blood cell disorders
    Burkitt lymphoma, 139
    cyclic neutropenia (cyclic hematopoiesis),
        136, 137
    Langerhans' cell histiocytosis, 140
    leukemia, 137, 138
    lymphoma, 139
World Health Organization (WHO), 127

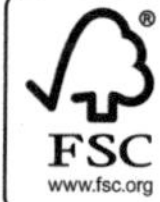